Don't Believe, What You Think

Werner Gross

Don't Believe, What You Think

Sense and Nonsense of Religion and Religiosity

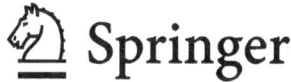

Werner Gross
Psychologische Praxis
Gelnhausen, Germany

ISBN 978-3-662-70877-4   ISBN 978-3-662-70878-1   (eBook)
https://doi.org/10.1007/978-3-662-70878-1

Translation from the German language edition: "Meinetwegen – nenn es Gott" by Werner Gross, © Der/die Herausgeber bzw. der/die Autor(en), exklusiv lizenziert an Springer-Verlag GmbH, DE, ein Teil von Springer Nature 2024. Published by Springer Berlin Heidelberg. All Rights Reserved.

This book is a translation of the original German edition "Meinetwegen – nenn es Gott" by Werner Gross, published by Springer-Verlag GmbH, DE in 2024. The translation was done with the help of an artificial intelligence machine translation tool. A subsequent human revision was done primarily in terms of content, so that the book will read stylistically differently from a conventional translation. Springer Nature works continuously to further the development of tools for the production of books and on the related technologies to support the authors.

© The Editor(s) (if applicable) and The Author(s), under exclusive license to Springer-Verlag GmbH, DE, part of Springer Nature 2025

This work is subject to copyright. All rights are solely and exclusively licensed by the Publisher, whether the whole or part of the material is concerned, specifically the rights of translation, reprinting, reuse of illustrations, recitation, broadcasting, reproduction on microfilms or in any other physical way, and transmission or information storage and retrieval, electronic adaptation, computer software, or by similar or dissimilar methodology now known or hereafter developed.
The use of general descriptive names, registered names, trademarks, service marks, etc. in this publication does not imply, even in the absence of a specific statement, that such names are exempt from the relevant protective laws and regulations and therefore free for general use.
The publisher, the authors and the editors are safe to assume that the advice and information in this book are believed to be true and accurate at the date of publication. Neither the publisher nor the authors or the editors give a warranty, expressed or implied, with respect to the material contained herein or for any errors or omissions that may have been made. The publisher remains neutral with regard to jurisdictional claims in published maps and institutional affiliations.

Cover illustration: © Michael Böhm/stock.adobe.com (Symbolbild mit Fotomodell)

This Springer imprint is published by the registered company Springer-Verlag GmbH, DE, part of Springer Nature.
The registered company address is: Heidelberger Platz 3, 14197 Berlin, Germany

If disposing of this product, please recycle the paper.

Preface

Being able to believe, can be a grace.
However, it is often our doubts that move us forward.

What do people believe in—and why actually? What benefit do they get from their religion? Is it different for Christians than for Buddhists, Muslims, or followers of nature religions? Does it matter whether we believe in the Christian "God the Father in Heaven" or in "Mother Earth" (Gaia)? Why are so many people flocking to the esoteric scene or the psycho market in search of meaning? What is truth for them? What is credible for them? What is sacred to atheists—what do they actually believe in? Generally—when is belief in religion(s) helpful—when does it become problematic?

This book is precisely about such questions. But not only that—the emotional processing also plays an important role: What happens intrapsychically when someone experiences their "enlightenment"? What happens in their psyche when someone loses their faith?—And what if they find a new faith?

Essentially, the topic is about the search for meaning in life: What do I orient myself by? What is a meaningful and a sensual life for me?

But somehow, the question of meaning is not quite so simple for us humans. If we are somewhat reflective, we can hardly escape the question of the meaning of our life. Does life have a meaning? Is it predetermined? And if not—can we give it a meaning?

Or are we humans perhaps "incurably religious", as the Polish philosopher Leszek Kolakowski thought? Because—whether we admit it or not—we are beings in search of meaning and try to make sense of why we are here, what we are supposed to and want to do in this world, in this life.

"When it storms and snows around the hut—that's the great time of religion," a wise person once said. Especially in crises, we often ask: Why is this happening to me—especially in the current situation? Is it coincidence? Or fate? Have we done something wrong—so are we to blame? Or is it even God's will?

For indeed, there is something greater and more powerful than us humans. Whether one calls it "Evolution", "Nature(laws)", "Energies", "(super)natural powers", "God/gods" or whatever else, is ultimately a question of the respective personal worldview. And despite all the differences between the individual religions, there are a whole range of similarities between them. However—which religion we end up with largely depends on the perspective that is prevalent in the respective culture and is passed on to us and the following generations through education. In most societies, the religious interpretation of this worldview is currently (still) predominant. Religions in particular like to speak of God—or at least of images of God and gods. And everyone has—more or less consciously—their subjective perspective on this. What can we know—what must we believe?

"Deluge of Meaning". In the market of freely floating systems of meaning, almost all claim that their truth is the only correct and genuine truth. Because in today's time of the deluge of meaning, where the eternal truths are dumped into our living rooms daily through the media, each individual can believe what they want—whether it is reflective and thoughtful or absurd and bizarre. Because even the belief in a—according to objective criteria—misguided system of meaning and worldview can be fulfilling and coherent for the person concerned and give them something.

Refuges from reality. In the attempt to unravel the mysteries of life, religions often oscillate between the ability to give people hope and the danger of producing illusions in them. But where does hope end—and where does illusion begin? The transition, unfortunately, is fluid. As a proverb so beautifully puts it: "Hope is a life jacket, but not a lifeboat." For many religions assume that God has a plan for each individual, for this world, and the universe. Others believe that God even intervenes in the life of each individual and that one can persuade him ("the dear God") to act in their favor through the right faith, appropriate prayers, rituals, services, or vows, etc. Thus, for some, religions are like refuges from the daily downpours, the banalities of life, and the cruelties of the present.

Others rather say "If God wills" (Islamic: "Inshallah") and submit to fate ("Kismet"). As if God would set it right: "Trust in God" was the term—when religion had a greater significance for many even in our latitudes. But it always revolved around humans and the human perspective. Because all religions seemingly elevate humans from their biological desolation. They give him the feeling of being sublime ("Crown of Creation")—or at least better than the predator.

Three Humiliations. "Man is the image of God"—this creed has been followed in the Christian cultural sphere over the past centuries. However, this view of the central role and uniqueness of man as the crown of divine creation had already received several setbacks from the sciences a long time ago:

For the ***first narcissistic injury*** to the special position of humans and the Earth in the cosmos dates back a few centuries:

In the 16th century, *Copernicus* indeed proved that it is not the sun that revolves around the earth (as had been thought until then), but rather the earth was demoted to a satellite of the sun and our home is by no means the center of the universe: A first severe insult to the anthropocentric fantasies of grandeur, as the medieval Christianity always invoked, proclaimed, and defended.

The ***second humiliation*** was taught to mankind by *Charles Darwin* in the 19th century. He viewed humans as the result of evolution and not at all as a unique and unchangeable crown of creation.

The ***third humiliation*** was finally inflicted on humans by *Sigmund Freud* and his psychoanalysis at the beginning of the 20th century: Freud proved that the individual human is not even "master in his own house", he is thus all too often at the mercy of his unconscious, his instinctiveness, and can only control himself consciously and voluntarily to a limited extent.

"Man is the crown of creation, if he knows that he is not," Carl Amery said, if man therefore does not assess himself in a megalomaniacal self-aggrandizement.

For despite these affronts, human hubris continues to celebrate again and again, wallowing in the old illusion of being at the top of evolution, and proclaiming the "Anthropocene", the human-made era. Religions contribute a significant part to this: "Subdue the earth," it says in the Bible after all.

If humans still consider themselves to be the image of God, perhaps it's worth taking a look in the mirror …

Interpretive authority and power of definition. On the one hand, the development of almost all cultures without the emergence and influence of religions is hardly conceivable. How they found (or dreamed) their beginnings and their images of God, religions were guiding stars for many centuries, by which first tribes and later entire peoples have aligned themselves (for more on this, see: Chap. 5: The past gods), by providing people with orientation in their respective time and cultural circle. Religions are therefore culturally mediated sets of rules that provide the framework and guideline for what is conveyed as appropriate in the respective culture, what is good and what is bad, what is right and what is wrong, what is allowed and what is forbidden.

For many centuries, religions held interpretive authority and the power to define in society and culture, in cities and communities, in clans, cliques, peer groups, and families. As a result, they (sometimes) provided each individual with help and support in difficult situations and times of need. For many, their faith was a "balm for the soul". Apart from that, religion was and still is the glue that holds many societies together. In earlier times, it was like this: Besides the political authorities (princes, counts, mayors, senate, councils), the most important people in a city or region were the doctors, the judges, the teachers—and the **priests.** The latter had—through their (supposed) connection to higher powers—a special role as open (or covert) advisors to the powerful (for more on this, see: Chap. 8: Gods, Prophets, Angels, Saints and Priests).

Appeals to the good in people. Despite all the differences between individual faiths,—understood benevolently—all religions (whether Christianity, Buddhism, Islam, or Judaism) are something like appeals to the good in people: So behaving well, decently, socially, justly, approaching one's own positive ideal self, rather than giving in to one's short-term instinctive egoism, is the implicit goal of most religions. In Islam, the "true Jihad" is also understood as the "holy war" against one's own short-term egoistic instincts.

The fact that the lived reality of religions is only limitedly identical to the ideal conceptions is another topic. Because fundamentally, this is about a cultivation process initiated by the religions, to orient oneself towards a good long-term (social and possibly even ecological) goal, instead of simply giving in to short-term egomaniacal satisfaction. "Like a drop in the ocean," as Buddhism says, we should fit into the course of the world. Whether one needs a god and/or a religious belief system for this, however, is another question. The fact that some climate activists ("Fridays for Future", "Extinction Rebellion", "Last Generation"…) no longer believe in the Christian "God the Father in Heaven", but rather have "Mother Earth" (Gaia) in view, may be something like their religious-ideological underpinning of their actions against the supposed "ecocide". Despair is usually good nourishment for illusions. Religion may be helpful (because it gives hope)—especially since there is something unquestionable (and thus providing security) in many religions, which is usually called God (or Allah, Jehovah, Brahman, Manitou…).

However, (religious) truth has become a perishable commodity today—and anyone who believes they possess this truth must reckon with its ever-decreasing half-life. Because eternal truths—as religions often claim for themselves—are becoming increasingly unbelievable for many—because it's a matter of opinion: some say one thing, others say another.

After all, religions deal with something invisible and have always oscillated between hope and illusion back and forth.

Narratives and Myths. Certainly, religions are more than narratives (stories) and myths that have been passed down over many generations. However, the crumbling reliability of religious faith has led to the churches losing the trust of many today. They have bound their members primarily with fear of hell and the devil for centuries, and where they held the dominant majority opinion, they kept the flock (also socio-psychologically) together with the fear of punishment for rule violations. In today's multi-option society, this only works to a very limited extent.

Twilight of the Gods. For religions are no longer what they once were. Due to globalization, all religions must undergo a process of relativization. Their respective monopolistic positions, which individual religions held for centuries in their respective regions, have crumbled in recent decades. They must (except perhaps in Afghanistan, Iran, and the Vatican) contend with competitors and rivals in a multipolar world on the market of worldviews. Therefore, religions have long since lost their innocence, and the credibility has often slipped away from them. More and more people—at least in our latitudes—are distancing themselves from religions—especially when they are preached in churches.

Loss of credibility. The problem is: credibility can be destroyed with a few wrong sentences or behaviors. The rebuilding of credibility requires (like a growth process in nature) usually a long time—and above all trust: And just as you can't squeeze the toothpaste back into the tube, you can't force Christian believers back into the churches. Because on the path of liberation from religious dogmas, many sacred cows have been slaughtered by now. And for quite a few today, it is something like a liberating redemption from the violence of gods and priests, from the fear of hellish punishments, if one no longer has to submit to the compulsion of religious dogmas and cultural traditions that dictate how one should live:

Today, especially young people are seeking, developing, and pursuing their own way of life. And these search movements are increasing. How do I want to live? What kind of meaning can I give to my life? Can I simply adopt the traditional religious offerings of meaning from religions? Or do I have to construct or search for my own meaning? For many, this search is open-ended: Sometimes you only know what you were looking for when you have found it.

While for centuries in this country believers were kept in the flock with the fear of hell (and the social pressure of the majority religion), this no longer works in today's multioptional society, where each individual has the choice between different systems of meaning. Whether influenced by Buddhism, linked with nature-religious practices or esoterically toned—believers want to be positively bound (if at all) today and no longer through threats and fear-mongering. Thus, the image of God in the Christian churches has changed quite dramatically over the last few decades—away from the punishing, threatening judge God, towards the merciful-loving God who accepts and understands: From the message of threat to the message of joy (for more on this see Chap. 6: Concepts of God).

Patchwork Religiosity. No question: Established religions can still contain many traces of meaning. Because these traditional systems of meaning of religions are still often unquestioningly adopted and passed on through education from generation to generation—even though many modern people currently do not discover this meaning in the major religions, but prefer to assemble their system of meaning themselves ("Patchwork Religiosity"). Because especially in the more developed regions of the world (Central Europe, USA, Japan), something is emerging that could be called "Twilight of Religions": Religion is only really important for a few—especially if it is church-dogmatic. While in the so-called "3rd world" even the Catholic Church, apart from the charismatically oriented Pentecostal communities, is still recording growth rates, the traditional religions and religious views in the highly civilized areas are of some relevance to at most a third of the population—with a downward trend: The sheep are leaving the shepherds. The dazzling power of religions has—at least in our latitudes—decreased and the demythologization of religions is in full swing. Religions may still have a calming effect on children—but fewer and fewer adolescents trust the religious beliefs.

Seekers of meaning. As mentioned: We humans are "seekers of meaning". Not only in crises do we want to understand why something happens to us and what sense it could possibly make. Why we are here, what we are supposed to do here (and want to do). Undoubtedly, therefore, the question of the meaning of life is good and justified—however, the preformed answers of religions are sufficient for fewer and fewer people: "Jesus is the answer—what was your question again?"

If they still have any significance for them, for many people today religions are something like the illusionary giant "TurTur" in Michael Ende's children's story "Jim Button and Luke the Engine Driver": The closer you look, the closer you get, the smaller the once immeasurably huge and inexplicable religions become in the fog of mysticism.

Off-the-rack worldviews. Religion elevates humans from their biological desolation. It gives them the feeling of being sublime ("crown of creation") and being better than the predator. Soberly considered, one could say: religions are systems of meaning with off-the-rack worldviews and images of humanity. And these traditional suits seem to fit fewer and fewer people today. More and more people—(e.g., "unbelievers", non-denominational, naturalists, rationalists, atheists, Marxists, etc.)—even claim that religions are something like "collective systems of madness", and in the worst case call believers "Religiot", who adhere to "conspiracy theories". Even the publisher of one of the formerly most important spiritual scene magazines "Connection", Wolf Sugata Schneider, writes in his circular 226 from 16.11.2022: "The so far most widespread conspiracy theory is that the world was created by an all-powerful old man in seven days, who lured us into believing in him by promising us his love."

Religions deal with something invisible. What one must not forget: All religions deal with and about something invisible—namely God. This is codified in the revelation scriptures that emerged centuries ago (Bible, Quran, Torah, Bhagavad Gita etc.), which were originally only orally transmitted and at some point written down and declared to be "God's Word" (more on this in Chap. 7: How the holy books became holy). And in the face of the invisible, they discuss different perspectives and interpretations of what one cannot see at all. But—the closer one looks, the greater the "questionability"—which means nothing else than questioning the worthiness: Dare to know ("Sapere aude").

I have always been amazed at how some people—be they theologians, priests, bishops, the Pope, or free-roaming prophets—have the courage to claim that they know what God wants …

How I came to the topic: The topic of religion and religiosity has occupied me for many years—what is good, helpful, and supportive about religions, but also what is problematic, unnatural, inhumane, and restrictive about them. I oscillate back and forth between these two poles—essentially since my childhood.

For my relationship with religion has always been tense and ambivalent. On the one hand, as a 10-year-old Catholic, I received the "holy communion" and was later also provided with the sacrament of "confirmation", even was—albeit very briefly—an "altar server" in the Catholic parish of St. Nazarius. On the other hand, I left the church in protest at 16 because I simply could no longer bear the narrowness and Catholic bigotry.

The ambivalence actually started much earlier. For example: As children, we were regularly sent to the Sunday (children's) early service, while our parents turned over in their warm bed and we had to go through the cold. The result: We did indeed leave the house, but rarely participated in the church service. Instead, we skipped the church visit and preferred to play "Old Maid" in the small alley next to the old Kolpinghaus, rather than listening to the priest's sermon. Even if it was with a guilty conscience. Until the mother then asked what the priest had preached about…

Nevertheless—or perhaps because of this—religion has always held a great fascination for me: As a journalist, I have produced a multitude of radio broadcasts and reports on various aspects of both the major churches and many different religious communities, subcultures, and sects. I still remember well my stay at the Cistercian Monastery Marienstatt in the Westerwald, where I was particularly impressed by the early morning chants ("Laudes") and prayers of the monks. But I also remember reports on Bhagwan disciples, Islamic Sufis, and Hare Krishnas, about psycho-sects ("Poisonous Paradises") and "mini-gurus".

Even before I became a psychologist, I was on the "hippie trip", hitchhiking all the way to India, spent a considerable amount of time in Benares (now: Varanasi), the holiest city of the Hindus, visited several ashrams and practiced yoga for many years. Later, I practiced Za-Zen in the Zendo against a white wall, sang Christian hymns, and performed the Sufis' "dhikr" and whirling dances a few times, chanted Manitu songs in sweat lodges with the Indians, and subjected myself to various esoteric practices—from gemstone therapy and Bach flowers to astrology, tantra, Watsu and Wata, rebirthing, all the way to Reiki and Native American ear candles.

The results were not final answers, but rather more questions that I was seeking answers to: What are they/we actually doing there? What is happening there? What's the point? What is the meaning? One could summarize the whole thing with the question: "Experienced a lot—but did you also understand something?"

Somehow, I never really understood God's will. And no one could really explain it to me. Or those who wanted to explain it to me were not credible to me. Thus, for me, religious faith oscillates between life help and delusion.

I rather agree with the old Jewish saying: "You are closer to God when you ask a question than when you give an answer" (for more on this, see Chap. 3: "Faith and Doubt).

"Religion can help, religion can harm." This quote begins an article in the "Journal for Religion and Worldview" (4/2023, p.284), published by the Protestant Central Office for Worldview Questions. And the article continues: "After the health-promoting effects of positive faith convictions and practices have been proven in the German-speaking area, reports are accumulating about the effects of toxic communities, religious violence, or spiritual abuse."

Psycho Market—Sects—Destructive Cults. In dealing with the two sides of religions, this ultimately led me, as a psychologist and psychotherapist (after some professional political struggles), to conduct a widely noticed BDP colloquium titled "Psycho Market—Sects—Destructive Cults" for the "Professional Association of German Psychologists" (BDP) on 24.01.1994 during the peak of the then "Scientology hysteria" (for more on this, see my book: "Psycho Market—Sects—Destructive Cults", Bonn 1998, 3rd edition). There was a multitude of articles, reports, and discussions on the topic: "How dangerous are sects? Why do people get involved? What can be done to get out? What do psychologists actually say about it?"—But other questions also arose: "What is actually the difference between a church and a sect? And what happened (and happens) in the churches? Is everything kosher there?", "What is the difference between belief and superstition?".

After I had developed the leaflet "What makes an alternative-spiritual group a problematic cult" for the BDP, the BDP working group "Psychomarket—Sects—Destructive Cults" was created in 1994 due to the many inquiries, which I led for over 23 years until 2017 (with several name changes: most recently it was called "Religion Psychology—Spirituality—Psychomarket"). In the over 60 mostly full-day meetings, we dealt with all possible topics:

- What is Shamanism?
- Effect of meditation on the brain.
- What characterizes dogmatism?
- What is spirituality?
- Religiously motivated suicide bombers.
- Exorcism in the Catholic Church—nowadays.
- What are enlightenment experiences?
- Psychotherapy and Buddhism …
- Etc.

Federal Enquete Commission "So-called Sects and Psycho-Groups". Ultimately, the working group was also one of the midwives for the Federal Enquete Commission "So-called Sects and Psycho-Groups", which met from 1996 to 1998 and for which I served as a scientific expert (for more on this, see the publication of the German Bundestag: "New religious and ideological communities and psycho-groups in the Federal Republic of Germany", Bonn 1998, German Bundestag).

And so I had the topic of religion and religiosity in view all my life. Sometimes with a more friendly-approachable attitude—sometimes from a more critical position.

"One begins their life as an arsonist
and ends it as a firefighter."
(Pitigrilli)

Heretic. That's why I have to admit it right at the beginning of this book: *I like heretics.* I am suspicious of people who unquestioningly (like a flock of sheep) follow a belief—regardless of whether it is Catholic, Protestant, Islamic, Buddhist, or atheistic.

> **For Consideration:** The german word "Ketzer" (heretic) is, incidentally, derived from "Cathars", a medieval sect whose members were annihilated, murdered, and mostly burned at the stake by Pope-loyal Catholics, particularly in France, primarily because they opposed the church's ostentation. "Kill them all, God will recognize his own," is said to have been exclaimed by Armaud-Amaury, a Catholic warlord during the Cathar persecution. This later became a battle cry of the Crusaders. The term "Cathars" originates from Greek and, incidentally, means "the Pure".

But there is an even more important reason why I like heretics: heretics have at least once thought about what they believe—or not. This cannot necessarily be said of most baptismal certificate believers (the herd), as many do not even know what they believe (should). Heretics have broken away from the herd and have—justified or not—sought their own path. Put kindly, one could also say it's about self-discovery and self-responsibility—if you will, the (re-)wilding of humans.

I myself do not fit well into a herd and do not want to be part of a herd—and I also do not need a shepherd who watches over me and tells me what is right and what is wrong. I prefer to think for myself, rather than unquestioningly adopting systems of meaning. *(That's why I have interspersed provocative "heretical objections" throughout the text—simply, so that this perspective is not completely lost.)*

Because that is a goal of this book: to demystify religions. It is about fundamental questions: What are religions actually? What benefits do they have? What damage can they cause? But it also deals with questions like: Is there such a thing as God or only images of God? If he exists: What can we say about him? Why do we search for meaning? Do biological roots of religiosity exist? Or is there even a "God gene"?

Beneficial Uncertainty. To avoid any misunderstanding: I am not trying to spoil people's positive experiences with religious faith. Quite the contrary: I want them to understand and integrate these experiences. Because miracles only exist for people who do not understand. When I understand, I am no longer overwhelmed, but can categorize what I have experienced.

Certainly, the book is still a provocation for some. And it is meant to be, because the word comes from Latin and means to provoke: I want to provoke people to find their own answers to questions of meaning. It is about—if you will—a "salutary uncertainty".

Thus, the book can also be understood as an appeal to think for oneself and to find and clarify one's own convictions on the subject of meaning—so to speak, to take a closer look at the stable of one's own positions (and possibly to clean it out). After all, everyone has a choice: The religion with which one has grown up does not have to accompany one for a lifetime (or even dominate and pursue): "Sapere aude", as Immanuel Kant formulated it: "Dare to use your own understanding" and to choose which worldview suits you.

It may be that the attentive reader of this book notices one or another contradiction in my explanations. This is not necessarily intended, but ultimately unavoidable in a work that is "work in progress". After all, it is also good to ask questions whose answer one does not (yet) know—simply because this is also a book for seekers, for skeptics, for the disappointed who have nothing more to do with outdated worldviews off the peg or the creatively absurd absurdities of the esoteric scene. It is also a book for heretics, an excursion for the relentless and against the dumbing down and exploitation by religion and belief—**but it is <u>not</u> a book against the search for meaning and faith in the sense of primal trust.** Besides, it is also a book for (and about) laughter in religious matters—for the "cosmic laughter". ("A god who can be insulted with blasphemous laughter cannot be a real god.")

It is important to note: I have no missionary ambitions and so this book does not aim to lead its readers to *any* particular faith or deter them from anything. It aims to help one find their own position on faith or—even better—develop it themselves. If someone absolutely needs an off-the-shelf system of meaning or even a dogmatic and rule-based religion, then that is also o.k. Ultimately, it is about plunging what is stupid and stupefying, or even tortures and terrorizes people, better into the abyss of oblivion. For this, there is occasionally the section: **For Reflection**

Of course, such a book also always reflects the current state of the author's engagement with the topic. As mentioned: It is "work in progress". So if you have suggestions, ideas, requests for additions or criticism, please feel free to contact me—preferably by email: pfo-mail@t-online.de. I look forward to your (even critical) feedback.

Internet: www.wernergross.com

Gelnhausen
Winter 2023/2024

Werner Gross

Contents

Part I What are Religions?

1	**The Janus-faced Nature of Religions**	**3**
	1.1 Benefits of Religion	4
	1.2 Thorn in the Flesh: Introject	5
	1.3 Globalization leads to the Relativization of Religions	5
	1.4 The Two Faces of Religions	5
	1.5 Blood Traces of Christianity	6
	1.6 Religious Wars Worldwide	6
	1.7 Forced Conversions	6
	1.8 Executions for "Waging War Against God"	7
	1.9 The Danger of Dogmatism and Fanaticism in all Religions	8
	1.10 Delusions of Grandeur and Luxurious Living	8
	1.11 Loss of Interpretive Authority	9
	1.12 Baptism Certificate and Submarine Christians	9
	1.13 Church Departures	10
	1.14 Questions of Meaning Remain	10
	References	11
2	**Man Thinks, (that) God Directs?**	**13**
	2.1 Helpful Illusions and Invented Truths	14
	2.2 Humans—a "Physiological Premature Birth"	15
	2.3 Belief Certainties	15
	2.4 Need for Orientation and Structure	16

	2.5	Adaptation Processes	16
	2.6	Ego-syntonic and Ego-dystonic	17
	2.7	Individuation vs. Societal Adaptation	17
	2.8	Worlds of Belief	18
	2.9	Excursus: James W. Fowler: Stages of Faith	18
	2.10	Script of Life: Fundamental Questions	19
	2.11	Questions of Meaning	19
	2.12	Religiosity	20
	2.13	Intrinsic and Extrinsic Religiosity	21
	2.14	Spirituality	22
	2.15	Teleology or Evolution?	22
	2.16	Is God an intelligent designer?	23
	References		24
3	**Faith and Doubt**		**27**
	3.1	Reality(ies)	28
	3.2	Three Truths	29
	3.3	Human—A Symbolizing Being	31
	3.4	What are Religions?	32
	3.5	Definitions of Religion	33
	3.6	Benefits of Religion	35
	3.7	Example: Buddhist Principles	36
	3.8	Problematic Aspects of Religion: Pious Inhumanity	37
	3.9	"Godless Priests?"	38
	3.10	Invisible Religion	38
	3.11	Belief—what is it?	39
	3.12	"faith" and "believe"	40
	3.13	Nihilism	41
	3.14	Serendipity	41
	References		42
4	**The Smaller (or More Confused) the Mind, the More Concrete must be the Image of God and Certainty**		**45**
	4.1	Do You Really know What You Believe (or should Believe)?	45
	4.2	Small Faith Test (Focus on Christianity)	45
	4.3	Don't believe Everything you think: Religious Neuroses	46
	4.4	Holy Simplicity or Religious Diversity?	47

	4.5	Typology of Believers and Their Attitude Towards Faith	47
		4.5.1 Gullible: "Unreflective-naive folk religion"	48
		4.5.2 Reflective believers: "Consciously and justifiably religious"	48
		4.5.3 Dogmatic know-it-alls: "You know it—but I know it better"	48
		4.5.4 Compulsive Fear believers: "Tormented by a guilty conscience"	49
		4.5.5 Skeptics, Rationalists, Scientists, Atheists, Naturalists: "I can't comment on that"	49
		4.5.6 Cynics: "Ironical Attitude"	49
		4.5.7 Religion and Church Haters: "Abolish the Churches!"	50
		4.5.8 Superficial: "I'm not Interested in Questions of Meaning—I don't care about religion"	50
		4.5.9 Agnostics: What can we really know?	50
	4.6	Fit: Who ends up in which Religious Group?	51
	References		51

Part II How Religions Became What They Are

5 The Past Gods: How Religions Originated—and where They have Evolved: From the Stone Age to Today   55

5.1 Where did the Gods come from?	56
5.2 From the Big Bang to the Emergence of Hominids	56
5.3 Genus Homo	57
5.4 Neanderthals and Homo Sapiens	58
5.5 Belief in the Stone Age	58
5.6 Origins of Consciousness	59
5.7 Burial Rituals	60
5.8 Grave Goods	60
5.9 Pre-religious Forms of Belief	60
5.10 Animism, Totemism, Shamanism	61
5.11 Belief in the Supernatural: Spirits and Gods	62
5.12 Cave Paintings	62
5.13 Sedentism	62
5.14 Emergence of Cities	63
5.15 Mesopotamia	64
5.16 Ancient Egypt	64

	5.17	Akhenaten	66
	5.18	Early India	67
	5.19	The Heavenly Abode of the Olympians: Greek Gods	67
	5.20	Roman Gods	69
	5.21	Christianity: Beginnings and Important Events	70
References			71

6 A Power Greater than Ourselves: Conceptions of God — 73
  6.1 Is there God/Gods or only Images of God? — 73
  6.2 The Multitude of Gods (Names) — 74
  6.3 Concepts of God — 75
  6.4 The Incarnation of God — 76
  6.5 God—Attempts at Definition — 77
  6.6 Advantages of a Personal God (Image) — 78
  6.7 Characteristics of God — 78
  6.8 What God has been used and misused for — 78
  6.9 Theodicy: Why does God allow so much suffering and injustice? — 79
  6.10 Reason and Faith—Proofs of God — 79
    6.10.1 Anselm of Canterbury (1033–1109) — 80
    6.10.2 Thomas Aquinas (1225–1274) — 80
    6.10.3 Nicholas of Cusa (1401–1464) — 80
    6.10.4 Thomas More (1478–1535) — 81
    6.10.5 René Descartes (1596–1650) — 81
    6.10.6 Blaise Pascal (1623–1662) — 81
    6.10.7 Baruch Spinoza (1632–1677) — 82
    6.10.8 Gottfried Wilhelm Leibniz (1646–1716) — 82
    6.10.9 Voltaire (Birth name: François-Marie Arouet, 1694–1778) — 82
    6.10.10 Immanuel Kant (1724–1804) — 83
    6.10.11 Georg Wilhelm Friedrich Hegel (1770–1831) — 83
    6.10.12 Arthur Schopenhauer (1788–1860) — 83
    6.10.13 Sören Kierkegaard (1813–1855) — 84
    6.10.14 Friedrich Nietzsche (1844–1900) — 84
    6.10.15 Bertrand Russell (1872–1970) — 84
    6.10.16 Karl Jaspers (Psychiatrist, Philosopher, 1883–1969) — 84
    6.10.17 Albert Camus (1913–1960) — 85
    6.10.18 Jean-Paul Sartre (1905–1980) — 85
    6.10.19 Ludwig Wittgenstein (1881–1951) — 85

	6.10.20	Hans Küng (1928–2021)	86
	6.10.21	Dorothee Sölle (1929–2003)	86
	6.10.22	Robert Spaemann (1927–2018)	87
	6.10.23	Kurt Gödel (1906–1978)	87
	6.10.24	Viktor Frankl (1905–1997): The Unconscious God	87
	6.10.25	Proofs of God: Conclusio	88
6.11		Belief and Knowledge: The Critical Voices	88
6.12		"World Soul" and "Sacred Matrix"	89
6.13		The Scientific Perspective	90
6.14		Conclusion	90
References			91

7 How the Holy Books became Holy: Their Origin and Function — 93

- 7.1 From the Visions of the Prophets to Canonization — 94
- 7.2 How and when was the Bible created? — 94
- 7.3 Torah, Talmud, and Tanakh: The Foundations of Jewish Faith — 96
- 7.4 Origin and Significance of the Quran — 98
- 7.5 Other Holy Books — 100
- References — 100

8 Gods, Prophets, Angels, Saints, and Priests: Who They are, What They Do, and What They Want — 103

- 8.1 Angels—Messengers between God and Man? — 103
- 8.2 Prophets: Proclaimers of Divine Truths — 105
- 8.3 How People Became (Made into) Gods — 106
- 8.4 God's Ground Crew — 106
- 8.5 The Dilemma between Freedom and Orientation: The Vertigo of Freedom — 107
- 8.6 The Longing for Credible Authorities — 108
- 8.7 Religious Authorities: Office Charisma and Personal Charisma — 108
- 8.8 Enthusiastic Youth for Faith: The Exploitation of Idealism — 109
- 8.9 Patronizing Care — 109
- 8.10 The Motivation to Become a Priest — 110
- 8.11 Religions' Approach to Sexuality — 111
- 8.12 "Purity Culture" and "True Love Waits" — 111

	8.13	Celibacy: Mandated Celibacy	112
	8.14	Blasphemy: Can one blaspheme God?	114
	8.15	Apocalypse—or: The Pleasure in the End of the World	114
	References		116
9	**Levels of Religion**		**119**
	9.1	Theological Level	120
	9.2	Philosophical Level	121
	9.3	Historical and Cultural Level	121
	9.4	Sociological Level	122
	9.5	Social Psychological Level	123
	9.6	Individual Psychological Level	123
	References		124

Part III The External and Internal Aspects of Religions

10	**Religious Organizations: From the Faith Community to the Sect to the Church**		**127**
	10.1	The Societal Role of Religious Communities	128
	10.2	Religious Flags in the Wind	129
	10.3	Counter-movements within the Church	130
	10.4	The Limited Tolerance of Religions	130
	10.5	The Infallibility of the Pope	131
	10.6	Religious Communities: Freedom and Democracy	131
	10.7	Churches and Sects	131
	10.8	Project World Ethos	132
	10.9	Caricature and Enemy Image	132
	10.10	Religion on the Internet	133
	References		133
11	**Religious Enlightenment Experiences and Altered States of Consciousness**		**135**
	11.1	"Homo Religiosus": Numinous Experiences	135
	11.2	Enlightenment in a Crash Course: "Illuminatio præcox"	136
	11.3	Mystical Traditions	138
	11.4	Unio Mystica: Union with God	139
	11.5	The Mystery of Consciousness	140

11.6	Altered States of Consciousness and Enlightenment Experiences	141
11.7	Triggers of Extraordinary States of Consciousness	142
11.8	Chemical and Pharmacological Triggers	142
11.9	Psychological Triggers	143
11.10	"God Helmet": Electromagnetic Triggers of Spiritual Feelings?	143
11.11	Does God Live in the Brain?	143
11.12	"God Module"	144
11.13	Neurotheology	144
11.14	Conclusion	144
References		145

12 What is Sacred to Me—or: Blessing is the Ability to Give Something You Don't Have Yourself — 147

12.1	The (Sometimes Hidden) Longing for the Sacred	148
12.2	Sacredness as an Intrapsychic Phenomenon	148
12.3	Group-forming Functions of Belief in Sacredness	149
12.4	Blessing: Support from Higher Powers	149
12.5	Types and Ways of Blessing	150
12.6	Sacraments and the Grace of God	150
12.7	Ordination	151
12.8	The Ridiculousness of the Holy	151
12.9	Can Everyone Bless?	151
12.10	Miracles?	152
12.11	Enjoying the Moment	153
References		153

Part IV The Light and Dark Sides of Religion

13 Humanistic and Authoritarian Religion: Salvation and Disaster Through Faith — 157

13.1	The Difference Between Authoritarian and Humanistic Religion	157
13.2	Authoritarian Religion: From Good News and Threats	158
13.3	Humanistic Religion	158
References		159

14 How Religion and Faith Become a Problematic Cult: Criteria for Sects — 161
- 14.1 Who Ends Up in Which Religious Community, Becomes at Home or Bound There? — 162
- 14.2 Seekers — 162
- 14.3 Disappointed — 162
- 14.4 Disoriented — 162
- 14.5 People in Acute Personal Crises — 163
- 14.6 People with Severe Mental Problems — 163
- 14.7 Fit — 163
- 14.8 Criteria for Assessing Spiritual Groups in the Esoteric Scene and Psycho Market — 164
  - 14.8.1 Ideology: Theory, Belief, Goals — 165
  - 14.8.2 The Central Figure: Leader, Master, Saint, Guru — 165
  - 14.8.3 Group Structure: Elite Community — 166
  - 14.8.4 Influence on the Member: Mind Control — 166
  - 14.8.5 Techniques for Personality Change — 167
  - 14.8.6 External Contacts and Dealing with Former Members and Critics — 167
- References — 168

15 Health-promoting and Disease-causing Religiosity — 169
- 15.1 Religion Makes You Healthy … — 170
- 15.2 Religion Makes You Sick … — 170
- 15.3 Perishing from Faith: Mental Illnesses Caused by Religion — 171
- References — 172

Part V Conclusion: Globalization - From Deluge to Flood of Meaning

16 Trust and Faith—What Really Helps (And What Harms) — 175
- 16.1 The Meaning of Crises — 175
- 16.2 No Power to Dogmas: Wisdom Instead of Belief — 176
- 16.3 Spiritual Wanderers — 177
- 16.4 Reason Against Dogmas — 178
- 16.5 Hope Instead of Illusion — 178
- References — 179

17	**Theses: Sense and Nonsense of Religion and Religiosity**		181
	17.1 World Explanation Systems		181
	17.2 Levels of Interpretation		181
	17.3 Origin of Religions		182
	17.4 God is a Human Idea		182
	17.5 Primal Trust vs. Faith		182
	17.6 Certainty and Dogmatism		182
	17.7 Subjectively and Objectively True		183
	17.8 What, How, and Why		183
	17.9 Knowledge and Belief		183
	17.10 Paradigm Shift: Time and Globalization		184
	17.11 Use and Abuse		184
	17.12 Gods and Wars		185
	17.13 Misuse and Demolition Houses		185
	17.14 Futility and Tolerance		185
	17.15 Distance to One's Own Worldview		185
	References		186
18	**Epilogue: With Both Feet Firmly in the Air**		187
	18.1 External Success and Inner Fulfillment		189
	18.2 Interchangeability of Religions		189
	18.3 Transnihilism		190
	18.4 Future of Religions: Digital Eternity?		191
	References		192
19	**Small Lexicon of Esoteric, Religious-spiritual and Philosophical Basic Terms**		193

Part I

What are Religions?

1

The Janus-faced Nature of Religions
The Holier the Festival, the Busier the Devil

> **Summary**
>
> This chapter deals with the *meaning* (i.e., the positive aspects that religions can have for each individual and society), but also with the *problematic aspects*, i.e., the dangers and nonsense that religions and exaggerated religious views and lifestyles can bring. Because religions always walk a tightrope between giving hope and the danger of producing illusions. It is certainly positive to give people the hope that life has a meaning (or at least one can give it a meaning). Anyone can also (if they see their life as meaningful and develop appropriate resilience) endure difficult and seemingly hopeless situations and grow from them. However, it becomes problematic and illusory when a religious worldview tempts one to solve worldly problems with religious practices.

*"The truth sometimes goes under –
but it does not die."*

Humans are probably the only creatures that know they will die someday (in the future). Other creatures live in a kind of eternal present. They may have vague feelings about their past, but probably no view of the (long-term) future. And here begins an important distinction between humans and animals: We humans have something called consciousness, for which there are various definitions, but essentially no one knows exactly what it is. Externally, it is certainly related to our ability to distinguish between past and future, to learn from the past for the future, to analyze, understand and predict complex issues in the long term, and to develop theories that are far removed from direct sensory reality and point to the distant future in their complexity. Not without reason do we nowadays speak more of the psyche and the former term soul is used less and less.

In the past, the **vegetative soul** of plants was distinguished from the **animal soul** of animals and the **human soul**, which was considered immortal and had a connection to the **world soul** (spirit, Ruach, Pneuma), which pervaded the entire cosmos in a subtle way. In more recent times, the question has rather been a scientific-neurological one. How does the brain actually make the soul? And how does the soul make God?

It may therefore make sense for people to erect meta-systems (laws, systems of meaning, religions) above themselves (or recognize them as natural laws) that they then no longer question (because the power that seems to be represented in them is wise, just, overpowering, etc.). If one is religiously oriented, one can call this "God".

"Who created God?", asked Stephen Hawking, who, alongside Albert Einstein, is probably the most famous physicist of modern times. He was already called the "century genius" before he died in 2018, being more or less immobile in a wheelchair due to ALS and only able to speak through a machine. He gave a simple answer to the above question: ***"Man."***

And this is where the whole dilemma begins: Did God create us or did we create God? Does God exist or only images of God? What can we really say about him? If he exists at all. In this sense, religions can be seen—superficially—as models of thought according to which people (more or less consciously) align their lives.

1.1 Benefits of Religion

No question: For true believers, religious ideas (belief in God or a superhuman energy) and spiritual practices (prayers, services, meditations) are helpful and supportive. For unbelievers, they are illusions. If they are well-disposed, they at least accept that the illusions are helpful for the believers. If not, they consider them to be (in the worst case dangerous) fantasies of "religiots".

Belonging to a religious community in which one has grown up is ambivalent for many today: On the one hand, one is born into a religion, has absorbed it with mother's milk, so to speak, and integrated it more or less well into one's own life over the course of life. On the other hand, the **"patronizing care"**, which is common in many religious organizations, is why many members distance themselves internally (or externally) from the religious community.

1.2 Thorn in the Flesh: Introject

On the other hand, there is much disappointment about what has happened and continues to happen in the name of, for example, Christianity: from the Crusades and witch burnings in the Middle Ages to child abuse today. This sticks in many people's throats and leads to an inner ambivalence and thus a distance from religious representatives, their know-it-all attitudes, and their repetitive old answers to the current problems of this world: "Jesus is the answer—what was your question again?" It is the many unanswered questions and the missing apologies from the church leaders, like a "thorn in the flesh," that festers in many believers and leads to this inner ambivalence. In psychotherapy, this is called an "introject", something that cannot be understood, accepted, and integrated.

1.3 Globalization leads to the Relativization of Religions

Due to globalization, religions must accept a relativization. Their monopoly position, which they had for centuries in individual regions, has crumbled in recent decades. They must deal with competitors and rivals in a multipolar world on the market of worldviews. The binding of members through fear of hell, death, and the devil only works to a very limited extent, because these—if they manage to break away—simply turn to another system of meaning.

1.4 The Two Faces of Religions

All Abrahamic religions (Judaism, Christianity, Islam) demand virtuous behavior and warn against sin: The true believers are rewarded by going to heaven, or punished by eternal damnation in hell. Here in particular, the Janus-faced nature of all religions—of whatever faith—is revealed: on the one hand, the bright, joyful or piously humble face of religions, which aligns itself with the guiding star of good faith and promises true believers a life in paradise, on the other hand, the fanatical and egotistical know-it-all shadow, which is based on the truth of the only possible religious worldview and insists on implementing the only possible world salvation plan, which must be implemented missionarily—no matter the cost: And if you are not willing, I need force.

1.5 Blood Traces of Christianity

Not only since the abuse allegations of recent years and decades have the Christian churches lost their halo. Because the halo has been crumbling for a long time. From the Crusades in the Middle Ages to today, the many instigated "holy wars" of Christianity and Islam, a trail of blood is drawn: In the name of religions, a lot of harm was also done on their path of missionizing the world. And not just today and in recent decades. The history of religions is unfortunately also a bloodthirsty history of torture and torment, of witch burnings, "auto-da-fés" (pronouncements of the Inquisition), of lynch law, murder, and manslaughter. And here, too, the enduring power of Christian priests, bishops, and popes—or in other religions the gurus, Brahmins, mullahs, or shamans (for more on this see Chap. 8: Gods, Prophets; Angels, Saints, and Priests). Because not least, the different religions are also the cause of many (faith) wars in the name of the respective religion: When the gods (or ideas of God) argue, in the worst case, entire nations wage wars against each other.

1.6 Religious Wars Worldwide

But not only in our latitudes have there been and are there religious wars: It is only a few years ago that even in the name of Buddhism, which is praised here in the West as so peaceful, the ethnic group of the Islamic Rohingya in far-eastern Myanmar was tortured, persecuted, and murdered. Their villages were set on fire, they were driven out of Myanmar by the Buddhist rulers to Bangladesh, countless women were raped, and many were killed. The same applies to Africa, where Islamist warriors from "Boko Haram" in Nigeria and "al-Shabaab militias" in Somalia repeatedly commit massacres on the civilian population, kidnap entire school classes, enslave and forcibly convert them. Not to forget the ignominious end of the so-called "Islamic State" (IS) in the Middle East.

1.7 Forced Conversions

Regardless, forced conversions of the defeated have always been part of cultural-religious subjugation, when countries were invaded, enslaved, plundered, and oppressed in the name of the respective missionary faith. And not only in Europe: In Africa and Asia as well as in Australia and America. And it's not as long ago as we might think: To this day, this is an issue among the Australian Aborigines and the indigenous peoples in Canada and the USA, where entire generations of native peoples were forcibly indoctrinated into the Christian faith in boarding schools—if they were not even killed or entire ethnic groups were exterminated in the name of religion. The tenor "Who converts, nothing happens to him" could rarely be relied upon. Sometimes, as a convert, one was simply treated and classified as a second-class human being, while the established believers posed as know-it-all master races in the name of their religion.

Pope Francis' attempt in July 2022 to apologize to the Canadian Indians for the abuse and many mistreatments and neglects of indigenous children since the mid-19th century is a start. But there is still so much to do …

1.8   Executions for "Waging War Against God"

The not infrequently found megalomania of religious leaders, that they have a direct line to (their) God, is exemplified in the following process: "War against God", with this justification, the indictment of the Iranian Shiite mullah regime against various participants of the protests (against the religiously justified obligation to wear the headscarf in such a way that no hair is visible) was titled—coupled with the threat to even impose the death penalty for it. And on December 8, 2022, the first of several demonstrators was indeed executed in Iran for "waging war against God". Since then, several people have been executed on flimsy grounds in the name of Islam. Unfortunately, they will probably not be the last—because a not insignificant number of demonstrators are still sitting in the death cells of the Evin prison in Tehran for this reason. One can only ask: Do these old bearded men really imagine that they know and execute the will of God/Allah?

It is only worse in the Islamic "God state" of Afghanistan, where the Taliban trample women's rights under the rules of Sharia. They are more or less confined to the house, are only allowed to move in public veiled (with a burka), are hardly allowed to pursue more demanding professions. Girls are no longer allowed to attend schools from the age of 16. As in our Middle Ages, hands are chopped off for theft. There are stonings for adultery and flogging for premarital sex. Morality guards control public life even more strictly than in Iran. And the so-called holy book "Quran", written 1,500 years ago, is the only guideline for everyday life. With the result that a large part of the population is starving, diseases are increasing, the economy is on the ground and medical care is disastrous. This is what it can be like when a strictly religious view takes over all power in a country.

*"One is all for religion,
until one has visited a truly religious country.
Afterwards one is grateful for sewage,
machines and a minimum wage."*
(Aldous Huxley)

1.9 The Danger of Dogmatism and Fanaticism in all Religions

Even if these are certainly extreme forms of religiosity—the real question is: Is the danger of fanaticism and dogmatism inherent in all religions—including Christian ones?

When taken to the extreme, the faith that alone brings salvation can lead to dogmatism, fundamentalism, fanaticism, and in the worst case, terrorism. For the womb is still fertile from which all this crawled—as is shown to this day by the recurring knife attacks, car attacks, and suicide bombings by both Shiite and Sunni Islamists here with us. But this kind of religiously motivated armed conflict was not only found in Islam, but also within the Christian religion, if one thinks of conflicts between Catholics and Protestants in Northern Ireland ("Bloody Sunday"). The situation in Israel and the disputes between Orthodox and liberal-oriented Jews also show how quickly religious fanaticism can lead to violent conflicts.

One could say that these are exaggerated misinterpretations of inherently peaceful religions by extremists who want to implement their religious world-saving plans with fire and sword. Cynically one could say: "The brighter the light, the darker the shadow", or: "The holier the feast, the busier the devil." Some time ago, a Protestant clergyman told me: "Religion is also capable of perversion" (for more on this see Chap. 13: Humanistic and Authoritarian Religion).

1.10 Delusions of Grandeur and Luxurious Living

It also fits that Kyrill I, the head of the Russian Orthodox Church and Patriarch of Moscow and Russia, not only blessed and supported Russia's war of aggression against Ukraine at the beginning of 2022 ("Military service is a manifestation of charity"), but also promoted Putin's personality cult, his delusions of grandeur, and a linkage of state and church interests—not to mention his own luxurious lifestyle.

However, the luxurious lifestyle is not a privilege of Orthodox bishops in distant Moscow. The former Bishop of Limburg, Tebartz-van Elst, had budgeted a whopping 31 million euros from church tax funds for his bishop's residence directly next to the cathedral—including a gold-plated designer bathtub for 15,000 euros, a conference table for 25,000 euros, and a garden that is said to have cost over three-quarters of a million.

But the other bishops (not only in Germany) also live well with the funds of the faithful and do not exactly live in Spartan-sparse conditions—as they often demand from their church members.

And some of them come into the crosshairs of the media or the public prosecutor's office—not only because of their handling of money. The Archbishop of Cologne and Cardinal Rainer Maria Woelki, for example, is repeatedly criticized for his handling of the issue of sexual abuse in the Catholic Church. Because of the same issue, the Bishop of Osnabrück, Franz-Josef Bode, even resigned in March 2023.

These are just a few examples and backgrounds for the loss of trust in the established churches. The large faith organizations have long lost their role as the defining authority (i.e., what is right and what is wrong) for most people. Ironically, one could say: "Whoever rises higher than he should, falls deeper than he wanted."

1.11 Loss of Interpretive Authority

Even though we fortunately do not currently have to endure open religious wars here in Europe—the struggle for the (only) correct worldview continues to smolder under the surface—dogmatism and fanaticism are always just a breath away in religions. And in this subtle struggle, the two major churches have long lost their interpretive authority and defining power in this field. Thus, anti-clericalism is increasing not only in this country but also in the general public. In sociology, this is called "Shifting Baselines", the change in basic reference values.

1.12 Baptism Certificate and Submarine Christians

Far more than a third of the population wants nothing more to do with the churches and does not pay church taxes. Just about a sixth of the total population in Germany (about 17%) are considered highly integrated church members (weekly church attendance, sacraments, confession, etc.) The rest are "baptism certificate" or "submarine Christians", who only show up in church at Easter and Christmas at most.

1.13 Church Departures

There is only one God in our midst—but fewer and fewer believe in him. Because the number of unbelievers seems to be constantly increasing: According to a survey by the Peace Dialogue Foundation, 61% of Germans consider religion to be "not important" or "not at all important" (Stern v. 29.12.22, p. 67).

Every year in Germany, currently between 600,000 and 800,000 members leave the two major churches. Dissatisfaction with the church institution (2021: 51.9%) is at the forefront for both denominations. There are slight differences in the reasons for leaving among former Catholics—there it is probably mainly the unbelievability of the church and the church leaders. For the former Protestants, an equally important reason is probably the evasion of church tax.

In the Bertelsmann Religion Monitor titled "The Future of the Churches—Between Loss of Significance and Reorientation in a Diverse Society", whose initial evaluation was published in December 2022, not much good is shown for the two major churches: Not only are the numbers of those who have already left the church very high, but also those willing to leave are at a record level. Thus, a further erosion of church socialization is expected. Many people nowadays live more by the motto "You can believe even without the church" (for more on this see Chap. 8: Gods, Prophets, Angels, Saints and Priests).

1.14 Questions of Meaning Remain

Ultimately, this is the background why the esoteric scene and the psycho market are still booming: Because they are disappointed with the established authorities, many turn to the free market of worldviews—simply because the questions about the meaning of life continue to exist. Only people are increasingly looking for the answers not from the established institutions, but believe they can find the answers in the freely floating worldview market between nature religions, esoteric practices, astrology, gemstone therapy, and Reiki.

References

Albus, Michael: Kirche nach dem Infarkt, Gütersloh 2007 (Gütersloher Verlagshaus)
Blume, Michael: Rückzug oder Kreuzzug? Ostfildern 2021 (Patmos)
Buggle, Franz: Denn sie wissen nicht, was sie glauben, Aschaffenburg 2004 (alibri)
Barth, Hans-Martin: Konfessionslos glücklich, Gütersloh 2013 (Gütersloher Verlagshaus)
Drobinski, Matthias: Kirche, Macht und Geld, Gütersloh 2013 (Gütersloher Verlagshaus)
Holl, Adolf: Im Keller des Heiligtums, Stuttgart 1991 (Kreuz)
Jaeger, Lars: Die Neuentdeckung der Welt, Berlin/Heidelberg 2022 (Springer)
Kermani, Navid: Ungläubiges Staunen – Über das Christentum, München 2015 (Beck)
Murken, Sebastian (Eds.): Ohne Gott leben, Marburg 2008 (Diagonal)
Ranke-Heinemann, Uta: Eunuchen für ein Himmelreich, München 2003 (Heyne)
Ranke-Heinemann, Uta: Nein und Amen, München 2002 (Heyne)
Rice, David: Kirche ohne Priester, München 1991 (Bertelsmann)
Schnepper, Arndt: Zankäpfel der Kirche Wuppertal 2007 (R. Brockhaus)
Trubach, Horst (Eds.): Was glauben die anderen?, Gütersloh 1993 (Gütersloher Verlagshaus)
VELKD Reller, Horst (Eds.): Handbuch religiöse Gemeinschaften, Gütersloh 1993, 4th edn. (Gütersloher Verlagshaus)
Wolf, Hans-Jürgen: Sünden der Kirche, Hamburg 1998 (Nicol)

Left

„Gefährlicher Glaube" – Betrachtungen über die Esoterik-Szene (deutschlandfunkkultur.de) (Stand: 16.09.23)
Kirche und Krieg: Gewalt im Namen Gottes? – ServusTV (Stand: 16.09.23)
Neue Studie offenbart Gründe für Kirchenaustritte – DOMRADIO.DE (Stand: 16.09.23)
Die unkomfortable Lage der Kirchenkritik: Zwischen den Fronten (herder.de) (Stand: 16.09.23)

2

Man Thinks, (that) God Directs?
Religiosity: The Emergence of the Intrapsychic meaning of Religion

> **Summary**
>
> This chapter discusses the individual, psychological perspective on each person's respective faith—why we need it and how it develops. It is about basic trust versus basic mistrust. What is religion to me? What is faith to me? Where does it help? Where does it hinder? What is God to me—if he exists for me? How much responsibility can I delegate to a higher power? Where is faith a delegation of responsibility? And how or by what does faith support me? This is what this chapter is about.

*"I did not know,
what I was looking for,
before I found it."*

The writer Charles Baudelaire said: "Man is a worshiping animal." And especially when despair and hopelessness prevail, some people become (again) believers. Especially when people's knees are shaking with fear, when they are overcome by despair, meaninglessness, the "cosmic shudder", when they no longer know what to do, then the religious primal images and primal mechanisms learned in childhood emerge: Suddenly, atheists start praying again, trying to negotiate with God after a cancer, AIDS or other life-threatening diagnosis, whom they had until recently considered the result of a delusional madness system of "religiot".

Are we doomed to hope in our primal longing for security? A true believer often becomes one out of despair. After all, our consciousness has been formed to a considerable extent by pain—simply because until then automated-unconscious processes simply did not lead to the desired results. Because it is simply hard for us humans to bear not knowing where we come from, why we are here, what we are supposed to do here and where we are going. This is probably an important reason why religions have developed (or were invented). It probably belongs to the "Conditio Humana", i.e. the conditions or circumstances of being human or the nature of man.

Similarly, it is not easy for many to bear that humans are supposed to be just products of chance (as many atheists believe), dispensable, interchangeable, meaningless. The term individual comes from the word meaning "indivisible". And as an indivisible individual, man—especially in difficult phases of life—is in search of a coherent interpretation and world explanation pattern.

2.1 Helpful Illusions and Invented Truths

Psychological processes are not exactly simple. They help us cope with the complexity of life. Therefore, it is worth unraveling them: Perceiving the world with our sensory organs, sorting and evaluating these experiences, forming internal representations of them, remembering and linking them with other experiences, comparing them and drawing the right conclusions from them is the goal. It is equally important to react appropriately externally, e.g. to plan a project, to make the right decisions in order to be able to act successfully—all this is highly complex. It gets even more complicated when it comes to religions.

Many people still prefer to believe in the understandable, tangible lie than the unbelievable truth. In this sense, religions may be just invented truths. But are religions then perhaps—especially in times of crisis—"helpful illusions? After all, religions have probably arisen to a considerable extent out of need and despair. And they have become so significant—because people were not able to understand and control the superhuman forces of nature, because they were and are at their mercy (for more on this see Chap. 5: "The past gods"). On the other hand, religions are consolations for those who do not cope well with the horror or banality of a meaningless and senseless life. Miracles only exist for people who do not understand.

One thing is clear: The preconceived beliefs and theories of religions must not contradict the findings of the hard laws of nature and the social sciences.

> **Heresy Objection** The ethical principles of the major world religions are (even if often only in theory) usually oriented towards human rights and make sense. The actual contents of faith, however, are more or less nonsense and produce magical views and world images.

2.2 Humans—a "Physiological Premature Birth"

A small developmental psychological excursion with a view to each individual:

We are all thrown into this world—toothless, wordless, and aimless. Delivered and unable to live alone in the first years, we are highly dependent. Because we—unlike most creatures in this world—are basically born very unfinished, we are "physiological premature births". Therefore, we (even more than all other living beings) need a "social womb" to grow up physically and mentally healthy. The first adaptation and education processes start here—with all the peculiarities of our parents and other socialization instances (kindergarten, school, training)—ultimately our culture. We are not talking about the development of the soul at this point.

We find the first sense of life in survival—which means first of all: drinking, eating, and being accepted, loved, and caressed in warmth—and in well-being.

2.3 Belief Certainties

It is the missing (or rudimentary developed) instinctual certainty (which is still present in most animals) that leads humans to mitigate their existential insecurity by wanting to have "belief certainties". Since we are the aforementioned physiological premature births with a large and complex brain, we need support from other people for much longer than other living beings in this world. However, the others are not necessarily very interested in us finding ourselves ("our thing") and really developing our potential freedom. Thus, it is not easy to gradually find our own position in the different phases of life and to consciously use something like our "free will" and to deal appropriately with the "dizziness of freedom" (Kierkegaard).

That's why there is this (more or less conscious) desire for meaning, for clarity, security, and unambiguity, which we find in religions or other systems of meaning (or believe to find). In the worst case, it is the dull and fear-tinted certainty of believers, where they swallow the fish along with all the bones. But: Maybe belief certainty is just the high art of graciously granted self-deception—and this applies to religious people perhaps just as much as to atheists.

2.4 Need for Orientation and Structure

Because apparently there is an inherent human tendency to want to understand oneself, others, and the world and to ask—in contrast to (other) living beings:

- Who am I?
- What am I doing here?
- What do I want here?
- Where do I come from?
- Where am I going?
- What is the meaning of all this?

And when we humans grow up, we first have this need for orientation and structure from the outside—and for explanation and evaluation of the impressions of the world. What is right, what is wrong? What should I do—and what should I better leave? And this is of course different in the toddler phase than in school time or puberty and adulthood. Not to mention that it is also assessed and evaluated very differently from culture to culture.

However—most people often take care of the question of meaning quite late. Sometimes it takes until retirement age to ask: Is that all there is? What have I done with my lifetime? Where have I really lived myself—and where have I let myself be lived by external demands? Have I just grown old in years or have I understood the world and the meaning (at least a little bit)? Have I just grown old in years or have I become wise?

2.5 Adaptation Processes

And for every developmental, growth, maturation, and learning step, we pay on the psychological level, because it is also a culturally shaped adaptation process. Thus, we sacrifice a piece of our original (archaic, perhaps also chaotic) identity on the path of cultivation, as we are shaped by parents, siblings and relatives, teachers, the media, ultimately society, and allow ourselves to be formed, bent (and also twisted). Thus, we grow up and align our potential inherent in us and are shaped by the environment.

2.6   Ego-syntonic and Ego-dystonic

Whether this goes well and we are one with it and identify with how we have become (psychologists call this "ego-syntonic"), or whether we struggle with it and rather have the feeling that it does not fit us at all, because it hurts and festers like a "thorn in the flesh" ("ego-dystonic"), this can vary greatly from person to person. Psychoanalysts used to call it "drive destiny", what we spend our lifetime with and where we end up. In the worst case, one might come to the realization that one has lived "the wrong life" because one has let oneself be too much influenced by the demands and expectations from outside.

> *"Actually, I am quite different —*
> *but unfortunately, I rarely get the chance."*
> *(Ödön von Horváth, writer)*

2.7   Individuation vs. Societal Adaptation

Instead of being supported in how we find our destiny ("individuation"), we are often used, needed, bent, exploited, abused by these demands. This is then kindly called "adaptation processes".

The background: In most societies, there are not many institutions that are interested in truly mature, adult, and independent people who know who they are, what is good for them, and what they want—simply because these people would not be so easily manipulated if they were more grounded in themselves.

The churches want—although they like to proclaim the opposite—above all *believers*, who unquestioningly adopt their more or less comprehensible belief system. The parties only want members and *voters* for their program, so they can implement their politics. The unions are looking for comrades-in-arms for their goals and the economy is looking for easily manipulable consumers and employees who are flexible to the point of unrecognizability ("people without properties"), who simply want what they should. And where does the individual with his question about the meaning of life remain?

2.8 Worlds of Belief

"Whoever believes in God,
needs no religion."
(Helmut Qualtinger)

No question: Until someone has really found his enduring faith, it takes a long time in the course of personal development—and a large part of it is not a conscious head decision, but full of emotional turbulences, confusions, and entanglements. Because in the development of the growing child, faith is initially pre-linguistic and consists mainly of trust. The "shine in the mother's eye", with which she looks at her child benevolently and lovingly, is (in addition to the appropriate physical care) the basis for this trust. Later, the world of belief of the child is shaped by his own wishes, feelings, projections, and fantasy ideas. In the Christian area, the "loving God with the long white beard" may then emerge. Only later, when the child's sense of reality increases, does the adolescent gradually understand the religious symbols and perhaps find his own critical position on them as a teenager—also through getting to know other viewpoints. In this sense, religions are invented truths adapted to the age of life. And it is often a long way to mature religiosity. If all goes well, the adult is able to critically question his own faith. It is about perceiving and tolerating that there are also other viewpoints and perspectives on it: The world is big enough after all, that everyone can be right (or wrong) in his own way.

2.9 Excursus: James W. Fowler: Stages of Faith

The American theologian James W. Fowler developed in his book "Stages of Faith" (Gütersloh 1991), based on the tradition of developmental psychologists Jean Piaget and Lawrence Kohlberg, a 6-stage psychological development theory of faith—regardless of which religion someone may belong to:

1. **Intuitive-projective faith**: After the child's basic trust has been established and consolidated in the first months of life, it develops its first own (also religious) ideas in the first years of life.
2. **Mythic-literal faith:** From about the 5th-7th year of life, the growing child can now also verbalize his/her faith, e.g. how he/she imagines God.
3. **Synthetic-conventional faith:** Slowly, the growing child develops his/her own faith identity (approx. 12–14 years). Many are dependent in this phase on

the "feedback" from "significant reference persons" mostly from their environment. Even later, only a few adults go beyond this stage.
4. **Individuating-reflective faith:** Own positions regarding faith are developed—even against the views of the environment.
5. **Conjunctive faith:** The complexity of different faith systems is perceived and the relativity of one's own faith is recognized, although this does not mean giving up one's own faith. Only a few adults reach this stage.
6. **Universal faith:** According to Fowler, even fewer people reach this stage (Mahatma Gandhi, Martin Luther King, Mother Teresa). These people are completely absorbed in their faith, without denying themselves.

2.10 Script of Life: Fundamental Questions

Both religion and philosophy are in search of the absolute truth. Who is the author of your life? Who wrote the script for it? Who is directing? Do you believe—you yourself? If so, by what criteria? Are they your genes? Is it fate? Or God? Is everything already predetermined—or do you have free will? And what do you base your decisions on when you can decide for yourself? What is your purpose in life?

2.11 Questions of Meaning

*"What does a fish know about the water,
in which it swims?
What does a believer know about the religion,
in which he believes?"*

The topic of the search for meaning is more widespread today than ever. Especially in uncertain times like today, the need for meaning of humans becomes apparent. He wants to know where he comes from, where he is going, what he is supposed to do here. Most want to understand who they are, how the world, the cosmos works, and whether they have a choice ("free will"). What they can know and what they must believe. In this context, finding meaning—if taken seriously—is often a lengthy process, like open-heart surgery—full of emotional irritations, full of risks with highs and lows, full of certainties and uncertainties. Because the central questions are only superficially easy to answer:

- What gives my life meaning?
- How do I give my life meaning?
- How do I deal with crises of meaning?
- From which sources do I draw meaning?

Whether I search for and find the meaning and the answers to the above questions in religions depends on a number of factors—e.g. the environment in which one grows up—the family, the village, the city, the culture. At some point, one is satisfied with it or reaches the limits and then the doubts begin—depending on how significant questions of meaning currently are for one. Especially in personal crises, the questions of meaning push into consciousness.

"Philosophy is,
when one thinks anyway."
(Odo Marquart)

In addition: Many are in search of a reason for hope—not only in times of crisis—some ask themselves banally: Where is the way to paradise? There is sometimes a stark difference between fearful skeptics and cheerful believers (more on this see Chap. 4: "The smaller (or more confused) the mind …). And in this context, religiosity and spirituality play a major role.

2.12 Religiosity

"People like to believe in something,
that elevates the banality of their existence."

One can say: Personal religiosity often arises from the desire for meaning, for an explanation of the world, and the attempt to trace unexplainable phenomena back to an understandable cause. Religiosity is subject to a complex neurobiological and psychological process, which, however, cannot yet be fully explained. What is certain, however, is that religiosity is **not** genetically anchored, as molecular biologist Dean Hamer claims in his book "The God Gene" (Munich 2006 Kösel). But most people probably carry within them the ability to develop a "transcendent sense". The philosopher and theologian Friedrich Schleiermacher (1768–1834) also finds in religiosity primarily the human "sense and taste for the infinite". However, there is no guarantee for a credible and exhaustive answer with lasting (eternal) value that also withstands the tests of reason.

One of my patients once formulated this inner ambivalence as follows: "God, you have done everything to make me despair of you and not believe in you. But I can't do it, I just can't lose my faith."

Not for nothing did the Apostle Paul supposedly say: "Faith is a scandal to reason." What may sound like an illusion to unbelievers is a certainty for believers. Perhaps one could say: Religions create dreams that warm.

Religions may also be an attempt to banish the invisible enemy of one's own insignificance and banality. Sociologists of religion claim that this sense of transcendence (for more on this see Chap. 19: Small Lexicon of Esoteric, Religious-Spiritual and Philosophical Basic Concepts) also offers evolutionary advantages—not only because it connects people in a religious community. For religious people believe in a transcendent power, greater than themselves, which—because it is above them—provides security and comfort and by which they can orient themselves.

This higher power, however, is not (completely) understandable, explainable, and provable and can appear very differently: For faith can refer to a **personal God** (Christ, Allah, Jehovah, Manitou …) or to a superhuman **force** or **energy,** that gives structure and meaning to life (e.g., Tao, Brahman, Evolution, Chi). Often associated with this is a reverence for the complexity and structure of life and the cosmos, in which many believers feel trustingly embedded as in the cathedrals of illusion. In modern parlance, this is called "serendipity", i.e., wisdom and intelligent luck (for more on this see Sect. 3.14). Also, (super-ego oriented) authority belief in this universal, celestial power is often associated with it. Highly religious people experience their existence as meaningful and align their experiences, thoughts, feelings, and actions according to their religiosity and try to implement this (more or less successfully) in everyday life. Some believers also have an intrinsic desire for "enlightenment" or "consciousness expansion" (for more on this see Chap. 11: Religious enlightenment experiences and altered states of consciousness).

2.13 Intrinsic and Extrinsic Religiosity

Religiosity is therefore usually about the highly individual experience of faith and practice of the respective religion, which focuses on the intrapsychic processing of the external belief system *("on the inner stage")*. This form is also called *intrinsic religiosity*.

In contrast, we speak of *extrinsic religiosity* when people become religious to gain personal advantages (e.g., belonging to an elite religious community, status, etc.).

Intrinsic religiosity is often associated with a high emotional charge (e.g., strong reactions to attacks) as it is often unconsciously linked to the core of the personality ("basic trust"). In different life phases, religiosity can have very different meanings.

Religiosity is primarily distinguished from

- *piety* (which strongly adheres to external dogmas),
- *hypocrisy* (only a religious facade) and
- *neurotic religiosity* (where religiosity is part of the mental illness).

Especially nowadays, people do not like to talk about religiosity—because the term is too often associated with the traditional major churches. Today, people prefer to speak of "spirituality".

2.14 Spirituality

The modern term spirituality is derived from the Latin word Spiritus (breath, spirit) or Spiro ("I breathe"). Spirituality is also a complex construct. Along with religiosity, spirituality also assumes that there is more than what we can perceive with our senses and explain with our minds (Transcendence). However, if there is a hereafter, it is definitely quite confusing.

In Christianity, spirituality is often equated with piety. However, spirituality is also lived completely independently of traditional religions—e.g., in the esoteric scene. Almost all spiritually oriented people have a "teleological view" of life, i.e., they find a predetermined meaning in life.

The psychologist of religion Sebastian Murken says about the difference between religiosity and spirituality: "Religion says: You shall, spirituality says: You may."

2.15 Teleology or Evolution?

"God does not play dice."
(Albert Einstein)

It is the old struggle between faith and knowledge: While from an evolutionary perspective it is assumed that developments in nature are undirected and playful (and depend on external conditions—sometimes also on chance) and can only be predicted to a limited extent where something evolves, in teleology it is assumed that all developments have a specific goal and purpose. Transferred to religions, *teleology* also means: God wanted to create man exactly as he is and has a special focus on him: "Sub specie aeternitatis"—from the perspective of eternity, as Spinoza formulated it.

> **Heresy Objection** Faith is fog, knowledge is clarity: The chance of evolution is our fate …

Charles Darwin, who significantly established the concept of *evolution*, found out that living beings adapt to their environment over generations and thus change their species. This can also lead to the emergence of new species. Supporters of evolution called this principle *"Survival of the fittest"*. Those who adapt only with difficulty (or not at all) run the risk that their species will become extinct. Some evolution-oriented people therefore believe that religions—because of the "dogma burden of their eternal truths"—will eventually become extinct.

2.16 Is God an intelligent designer?

In contrast to evolution, teleology postulates the purposefulness and goal-directedness not only of human action, but of nature as a whole. Teleological thus means being related to a goal or purpose and assumes a purpose. Teleology means that actions, things, and processes consistently proceed in a goal-oriented manner in their origin and development. What the goals consist of and who or what their cause is—whether a God, a creative principle or energy potential, or the human (Anthropomorphization = humanization)—has been hotly debated in philosophy, science, and theology since antiquity.

Especially in Bible-believing conservative-creationist circles in the USA, "Intelligent Design" is advocated and propagated, that is, that God made an intelligent design of the world and the universe, according to which all life develops preplanned evolves. Creationists take the creation of the world described in the Book of Genesis literally. The six days of creation and the day of rest each last 24 hours—the first week after the absolute beginning of time. The entire Bible is, according to creationist belief, a truthful, historical report. According to the creationists, the earth is therefore a maximum of 10,000 years old. Most often, however, an age of about 6,000 years is given.

The counter-position to this is that religions could indeed only be a byproduct of evolution, which will eventually disappear due to their dogmatic burden.

Food for thought And what do you believe?

"A blind man is a good guide in the dark of night.
During the day, one should rely on one's eyes."

References

Bor, Jan, Petersma, Errit: Illustrierte Geschichte der Philosophie, München 1997 (Scherz)
Currie, Ronald F.: Gott ist tot, München 2008 (Goldmann)
Frankl, Viktor E.: Die Sinnfrage in der Psychotherapie, München 1981 (Piper)
Federspiel, K., Lackinger-Karger, I.: Kursbuch Seele, Köln 1996 (Kiepenheuer + Witsch)
Fowler, James W.: Stufen des Glaubens, Gütersloh 1991 (Gütersloher Verlagshaus)
Grom, Bernhard: Religionspsychologie, München 1992 (Kösel)
Goldner, Colin: Psycho – Therapien zwischen Seriosität und Scharlatanerie, Augsburg 1997 (Pattloch)
Kakuska, Rainer (Eds.): Andere Wirklichkeiten – Die neue Konvergenz von Naturwissenschaften und spirituellen Traditionen, München 1984 (Dianus/Trikont)
Küng, Hans: Existiert Gott? Freiburg 2017 (Herder)
Lennox, John: Gott im Fadenkreuz, Witten 2013 (SCM-Brockhaus)
Moser, Tilmann: Gott auf der Couch, Gütersloh 2011 (Gütersloher Verlagshaus)
Moser, Tilmann: Gottesvergiftung, Frankfurt 1976 (Suhrkamp)
Schlette, Heinz Robert: Weltseele – Geschichte und Hermeneutik, Frankfurt 1993 (Knecht)
Sheldrake, R., Fox, M.: Die Seele ist ein Feld, München 1998 (O.W. Barth)
Utsch, M., Bonelli, R. M., Pfeifer, S.: Psychotherapie und Spiritualität, Berlin/Heidelberg 2014 (Springer)

Wilber, Ken: Naturwissenschaft und Religion, Frankfurt 1998 (Krüger)
Wiesenhütter, Eckart: Religion und Tiefenpsychologie, Gütersloh 1977 (Gütersloher Verlagshaus)
Wilber, Ken: Das Spektrum des Bewusstseins, Reinbek 1991 (Rowohlt)

Left

Der Mensch – eine physiologische Frühgeburt – weiterbildung-im-fernstudium.de (Stand: 18.9.2023)
Ich-Dystonie – DocCheck Flexikon (Stand: 18.9.2023)
Teleologie – Wikipedia (Stand: 18.9.2023)

3

Faith and Doubt

"You are Closer to God When You Ask a Question than When You give an Answer."

> **Summary**
>
> This chapter deals with the way in which one approaches the topic of religion and faith with appropriate doubt. Do I **thrive in faith** or do I **perish in faith**? It is good to start by asking a few naively stupid questions. What is reality—and what is (religious) truth? Is there the true religion? What can we know about God (or gods)? It is about the distinction between knowledge and belief: Do you still believe or do you already know?

"Only a few know,
how much you have to know,
to know,
how little you know."
(Werner Heisenberg, Physicist)

No question: There is reality—but can we really recognize it? Or more precisely—what of it can we recognize? What can we really know? And what do we have to believe? What is true for us? And: How much illusion does man need? These questions concern not only religions, but our entire attitude towards reality, towards reality.

"Reality,
reality
really wears a trout dress
And turns silently
and turns silently

After other realities."
(André Heller)

3.1 Reality(ies)

But what is real? In a banal sense of the word, one could say: What is real is what has an effect. Philosophically, reality is seen as the "in-itself-being", the "actual being", the "being in space and time", the "objective". In short, it is initially all that is directly perceptible in terms of facts. However, things also exist independently of our perception: The moon is still there even when no one is looking.

Let's start with the basics: We primarily perceive the world through our sensory organs (seeing, hearing, touching, smelling, tasting)—ideally in a holistic and undivided way. So it's about perceiving the outside world with our sensory organs (and of course also with what we humans have developed as technical devices to extend our senses). It is our task to categorize and evaluate these experiences. We should be able to form inner representations of them, remember them, and link them with other experiences in order to draw the right conclusions and follow up with appropriate actions. All of this is highly complex.

It gets even more complicated when it comes to religions, as this involves something not directly visible: God and gods are invisible after all. Because it's not just about knowledge, but also about belief. "Do you still believe—or do you already know?", the atheistically oriented Giordano-Bruno-Foundation formulates. But what do we really know with absolute, unquestionable certainty? And there are different views on this as well.

In constructivism, for example, it is assumed that every reality is constructed. For constructivists, there is no objective reality, but it is always constructed by the observer of a situation or state. So the question is not whether you are lying, but whether others believe you.

The well-known systemic therapist Paul Watzlawick believed that reality is the result of communication. He considers the idea that there is only one reality to be a problematic self-deception. And since there are many subjective realities for Watzlawick, he believes: "Everyone thinks that his reality is the real reality."

> "When a philosopher answers a question for me,
> I often no longer understand my question."

In order to be able to experience something in the here and now as present and real, we must merge memory (i.e., the past) and expectation (i.e., the future) in such a way that the current perception and interpretation becomes our own position. Because all people need and have (more or less consciously) a system of explaining the world, be it biological, naturalistic, philosophical, esoteric, or religious.

In social sciences, the term concept of reality is used to denote what people believe to be true and real and what they base their actions on. And there is a lot of opinion, but little understanding and knowledge.

"There is reality, and it is not to be shaken."
Truths, however,
namely opinions about the real expressed in words,
there are countless.
And each is as right as it is wrong."
(Hermann Hesse)

In this context, the terms reality and truth are often used synonymously in common language, although they can differ greatly: Reality points to something that is effective, while truth tries to recognize and interpret reality.

3.2 Three Truths

In summary, one can distinguish three types of truths:

1. **Subjective truths:** What I personally believe to be true.
2. **Objective truths:** What is objectively visible or recognizable and verifiable (e.g., with cameras or other instruments).
3. **Interpersonal truths:** What a group (e.g., a religious community) has agreed upon as being true.

Institutionalized religion often acts as if it were objective truth. However, religions can best be seen as **interpersonal truths**. For non-believers, religions may be an illusion. For believers, they are (inter-)**personal truth**—and thus (at least superficially) helpful and useful. Because one must believe in ideas for them to work (positively). They can also be harmful as illusions—but more on that later.

Truths—it seems—are many and they are subjective, interpersonal, and only rarely objective. Simply because personal interpretation and subjective meaning always play a role.—And truths are perishable. Some even speak of a "truth illusion": What is considered true today may be an illusion tomorrow. As Friedrich Nietzsche wrote: "Truth is an illusion without which a certain species could not survive."

> *"A lie has already run around the world three times,*
> *before the truth puts on its shoes."*
> (Mark Twain)

If someone is seeking the truth, they should not be shocked when they find it. Because religions are full of invented truths. However, there also seem to be truths that cannot be proven by scientific means and yet are true: Human knowledge is always only piecemeal. Because man knows little in essence, but believes that what he knows is the truth and that gives him the right to dictate to others and—in extreme cases—to kill them if they do not subscribe to his viewpoint, his belief.

The problem arises when knowledge is subordinated to belief and is distorted by belief, "because what cannot be, must not be": "The earth is the center of the universe." So it is not without danger when the church teacher Thomas Aquinas proclaims: "Philosophy is the handmaid of faith." Vulgo: Faith is more important than knowledge.

A few centuries earlier, the Apostle Paul is said to have said: "Faith is a scandal to reason." However, faith must not contradict reason. Because reason and will are good servants, but they are bad masters. So one can say: Faith is only limitedly explainable on a rational level.

"Man errs as long as he strives," Goethe lets Faust say in his famous religiously critical play. Because unlike religion, philosophy assumes the equality of good and evil. So—always consider that you could be wrong.

> *"Happy can he feel,*
> *who is able in the long term*
> *to believe, he understands the world."*

For Reflection Do you find the truth that makes you happy?

So there are the most diverse religious—sometimes also absurd—truths, which we will look at again and again. Here is, for example, one:

James Usher (1581–1656), highly respected Irish Anglican theologian, Archbishop of Armagh and Primate of Ireland, calculated from the life dates of biblical figures that God completed the creation of the world exactly on October 23, 4004 (BC) at 8 o'clock in the morning. Can this be true?

> **Heresy Objection** What should we believe? And where does the nonsense start? Should we really believe all that which has encountered certain people (who were later perhaps referred to as prophets or even as gods) a long time ago in their fantasies or fever dreams? And what was proclaimed as "eternal truths" in the so-called "holy books"?

3.3 Human—A Symbolizing Being

The human being is a constantly changing subject. As proven in various recent psychological studies, he/she does not have such a fixed "I", but is constantly changing: Today he/she is successful, tomorrow he/she fails. Sometimes he/she is a shining hero, sometimes a tragic figure. Sometimes he/she is sad, sometimes angry or joyfully excited, sometimes just funny. He/she is a wanderer between his/her emotional states. Sometimes he/she is also an observer, an uninvolved "witness" of what he/she does and what happens to him/her. And (almost) always he/she is so identified with this position that he/she thinks: This is exactly who I am, this is my core.

"Who am I—and if so, how many?" was a philosophical bestseller by Richard David Precht a few years ago, which dealt precisely with the questions of the core of personality, self-knowledge and self-image. Who (or what) is it that perceives something? Is there perhaps this constant core of identity, which some religions refer to as the soul? In depth psychological psychotherapy, a distinction is made between "I" and "self", with the self being seen as a kind of core of personality…

In our experience, it is particularly important to distinguish between what we perceive concretely and the way we interpret it. And our interpretation often happens in words and signs, i.e., symbols. The human being is an "animal symbolicum", a symbolizing animal that makes the world accessible to itself through symbols (words + signs), says the philosopher Ernst Cassirer. In concrete terms: We live and think primarily in words and symbols. And religions are a collection of symbols and words. And words create worlds—not just religious ones.

How important words can be is shown, for example, even in very simple terms that evoke completely different associations. Test for yourself:

> **For Reflection** What different associations and feelings do you have with the terms:
>
> - Religion**less** or religion**free**?
> - Suicide or voluntary death?

3.4 What are Religions?

*"Believing means
losing your mind,
to gain God."*
(Søren Kierkegaard)

On the sociological level, religion is a culturally mediated set of rules that dictates what is right and wrong in a society. Seen in this way, religions can—superficially—be described as models of thought according to which people (more or less consciously) align their lives.

It is not so long ago that the church prescribed to people how they should see people, the world and the cosmos: Only the Christian lives correctly and the earth is the center of the universe around which the entire cosmos revolves. Galileo Galilei, who saw it quite differently, had to recant, otherwise he would have ended up at the stake. Nevertheless, he said: "I do not feel obliged to believe that the same God who has endowed us with senses, reason, and intellect has intended us to forgo their use" (Galileo Galilei, 1564–1642).

And in this conflict we all stand—more or less consciously: We are supposed to see and interpret the world in a certain way that the religions dictate to us, even though we might interpret it quite differently ourselves. This is one (though not very important) reason why more and more people are distancing themselves from their religious views.

50 years ago, 96% of the population still belonged to a church. At that time, the proportion of people who belonged to *no* church was just 4%. By 2023, this had already risen to 40% who had left the church. If this continues, we will end up with what the Giordano Bruno Foundation calls the "Secular Decade": At some point, the majority of Germans will be "confession-free" (not without confession).

This is also the goal of the "Central Council of the Confession-Free", an association of several secular associations, which aim to represent the interests and rights of people who do not belong to any religious community. Because, although we are officially a secular state, the two major churches still have an immense influence on many political decisions: Whether it is about abortion, voluntary death, ethics teaching (instead of religious instruction) or special church labor law—everywhere the two major churches (more or less covertly) exert their influence.

3.5 Definitions of Religion

There are numerous attempts to define the term religion. The word religion originates from the Latin terms "religare" (to bind, to descend) or "relegere" (to read again, to reconsider, to conscientiously follow duties) or "religere" (to choose again). Often, religion is understood as something like "reconnection" and (primal) trust.

For many, religion is the belief in a supernatural power (in this country mostly God or Allah). Some understand religion as "worship of God" or even "fear of God".

Religions are not just enduring narratives, i.e., stories passed down from generation to generation. For some, they are the basis of their identity. What can be said is: How I assess religion and what significance it has for me depends to a large extent on the standpoint from which I view religion.

Non-believers assume that faith is only a real achievement when one believes in something that is quite unlikely or even nonsensical. In Islam, it is said: "Trust in Allah—but tie your camel's feet."

But what exactly is religion? How does it manifest itself? Does religion primarily manifest itself in certain obvious rituals (services, prayers, chants, meditations) or in certain sacred buildings (churches, temples, synagogues, mosques)? Is it what is represented and proclaimed by religious officials (priests, bishops, mullahs, gurus …)? Or is religion just something highly subjective, which everyone develops for themselves and then believes in?

> **For reflection** What is a credible religion for you? How do you determine it? What significance does it have for your life? What does religion do to you? Where, how, and in what actions does it manifest itself? What about it is positive—and what about it is problematic?

"Religions are like fireflies,
they need darkness,
to shine."
(Arthur Schopenhauer)

Excursion: The following narrative describes in an allegory the differences between "true religion" and a belief based on traditions, myths, and falsehoods. It is attributed to the founder of the Bektashi Sufi order, Haji Bektash (1209–1271).

The Story of the Holy Tomb

Long ago, there lived the son of a highly respected administrator of a holy tomb, which had become a true pilgrimage site for many believers. He was supposed to succeed his father at this holy pilgrimage site and thus have a good and comfortable life ahead of him.

But when he grew up, he decided to seek the truth and knowledge himself—wherever they might be found—even if "I find them in China".

With his father's blessing, he saddled his donkey and set out into the world.

In the many years of his wanderings, he visited various cities and countries: He visited Cairo, Damascus, and Aleppo, traversed Babylonia, the land between the two rivers, the Arabian desert, was in Samarkand and Bukhara, met several dervishes and was in several Tekkes of the various Sufi orders. When, after many years on the road, he was in the heights of the Hindu Kush mountains on his way towards Kashmir and Tibet, his donkey died due to the many hardships and because the air up there was so thin.

Since the donkey had been his only companion for many years and decades, accompanying him everywhere, he was very sad. Bent with pain and with a broken heart, he buried his companion under a simple mound of earth. Quietly meditating, with the high mountains above him and the mountain streams rushing into the valley below him, he spent his time at this crossroads of mountain roads, connecting Central Asia, India, and China with Persia, Turkmenistan, and Uzbekistan.

Soon, the traders and pilgrims noticed the solitary man who alternately mourned his loss and stared blankly down into the valley.

"It must be the grave of a saint," they whispered to each other. "If someone, who is probably himself a disciple of a saint, is so long and for weeks at a time given over to his pain and finds no relief."

When a rich man with his caravan passed by after a few months, he ordered a dome and a tomb to be built at the site. Other pilgrims terraced the mountainsides and planted fruits to support the maintenance of the holy tomb.

After some time, the fame of this new pilgrimage site with the silently mourning dervish spread throughout the region. When the father heard about it, he immediately set out for this new sanctified place.

When he arrived there, he was surprised to find that it was his son, and he asked him what had happened. The son told him (in a whisper) the story and said: "The pilgrims are so full of faith, love, and hope that I did not want to disappoint them by telling them the truth."

Then the father raised his hands to heaven and said: "My son, the tomb where you grew up was also created in the same way when my donkey gave up its spirit there more than thirty years ago."

3.6 Benefits of Religion

As we humans are creatures in search of meaning, religions elevate us above biological simplicity and provide comfort for the everyday downfalls of life. The basic idea of most religions is almost always idealistic. Their goal is usually to develop the good in humans. However, the implementation often falls short—simply because it is all too human even in many religious communities.

People project something into the gods, which they then follow. They thus surrender power to something greater (God) so that they can feel safe and secure. Especially the simple-minded have a god who protects them, for holy simplicity often contradicts religious diversity. Arno Backhaus, a Christian songwriter who likes to call himself an "E-fun-gelist" and "Missio-Narr", says: "God plays no role in my life. He is the director."

> *"Religion is a protest*
> *against the meaninglessness of events."*
> *(Martin P. Nilsson, Swedish historian)*

Another positive aspect of religions is that they develop structures for the inexplicabilities of life, that they provide hope and basic trust, and convey the feeling that not everything is explainable (and does not have to be). Because religions are world explanation systems that try to explain the invisible through visible symbols and words. They almost always contain a power greater than ourselves (usually God, or similar). They are systems of meaning that provide answers to philosophical questions of meaning. They thus structure unstructured situations and help to make the incomprehensible understandable.

> **For Reflection** How far does hope go—and when does illusion begin?

> *"He who has a 'why',*
> *can bear any 'how'."*
> *(Friedrich Nietzsche)*

The symbols, images, and metaphors of a religion serve to make understandable to people what is actually not (or only symbolically and very difficult) expressible in words. Because how can one communicate about something invisible without images and words?

Nevertheless: The ethical principles that all serious religions have in common are helpful for human coexistence.

3.7 Example: Buddhist Principles

In Buddhism, for example, there are the four great truths that believers should align their lives with:

1. Life is suffering
2. Suffering arises from desires
3. Desires can be overcome
4. The eightfold path to overcoming desires is:

   – Right view
   – Right intention
   – Right speech
   – Right action
   – Right livelihood
   – Right effort
   – Right mindfulness
   – Right concentration

Implemented in everyday life, these rules ("Silas") of Buddhism look like this:

- I will not cause harm to any living being.
- I strive not to hurt any being with my speech.
- I take nothing that is not given to me.
- I strive not to misuse any being in any way or to cause harm through my (sexual) behavior.
- I do not take any intoxicating substances.

So much for the theory—the implementation into everyday life practice is just as difficult for Buddhists as it is for Christians, in Judaism or in Islam.

Because many of these ethical principles can also be found, for example, in the Ten Commandments of Christianity or in other religious rule sets. Where these ethical principles differ between religions, they are more or less nonsense influenced by culture and the spirit of the times.

3.8 Problematic Aspects of Religion: Pious Inhumanity

Religions act as if they are wrinkle-free systems of meaning. Through their dogmas, they usually have static worldviews, which they only sometimes adapt to the spirit of the times. In this sense, religions are often mummified truths. Nowadays, the ashes are often worshipped rather than the fire being carried on.

They are also specialized in exploiting the idealism of their believers and satisfying the need for a magical explanation of the world. Religion is not magic. But unreflected faith can undoubtedly produce magical views.

Problematic for the off-the-shelf religious worldviews can be that believers are primarily bound by fear (e.g., of hell), that dogmatism, extremism, fanaticism—and in the worst case terrorism and religious war are the result. Because most religions carry within them the danger of becoming fanaticism through their dogmatism. This can also lead to what one could call "pious inhumanity". And it's not just about the sexual abuse of children by clerics. One only has to remember what was done in Christian children's homes by nuns, monks, priests, and believing supervisory and teaching staff.

Not infrequently, the pious divide humanity into believers (friend) and unbelievers (enemy). Their certainty of faith leads to the fact that the dogmas may not be questioned: Intrapsychically, they maintain themselves (because they are in a kind of "holy war") through the connection with their all-powerful believed God (and because they believe to execute God's will) sometimes for invulnerable. This invulnerability of the simple-minded goes hand in hand in the worst case with a kind of delusion of omnipotence. They give themselves religious permission based on their higher goal to dictate to other people how they should live, and if they do not obey, to imprison them or even slaughter them in the worst case. They often confuse faith content and basic trust: The smaller (or more confused) the mind, the more concrete the image of God must be.

> **Heresy Objection** Religions are the virtuous ghosts that lure us with illusions and terrorize us with fear.

Critical views of religion have been around for a long time: "Religion is socially sanctioned madness," some atheists say. And "Religion is pathology, not theology," Ludwig Feuerbach said 200 years ago—and: "Man is not God's work, God is man's work" (more on this see Chap. 6).

3.9 "Godless Priests?"

"Religion is curable," is the title of a book on the subject of faith by the former Catholic priest Josef Hochstrasser, who was later ordained a Reformed pastor in Switzerland. Subtitle: "From the perspective of an agnostic". Can such a thing work: a priest who is questioning his faith?

Apparently yes.

Perhaps a subjective experience from my psychotherapy practice:

When I think of the various Catholic, Protestant and otherwise religiously bound church officials I have had in psychotherapy, counseling or coaching over the many years, the proportion of agnostic (or even atheistic) priests who have doubted their faith—and sometimes even despaired of the "traditional religious chatter"—is quite high. We often talked about how they deal with the discrepancy of proclaiming religious truths to the community on the outside that they themselves no longer believed in. A church official once told me: "The higher you get in the middle church hierarchy, the greater the proportion of doubters, unbelievers and cynics. What some bishops preach to the sheep, he himself often no longer believes in." Ergo: The staff still believes in God. The rule has long been nihilistic.

> Another small scene that I observed in my direct environment with two of my friends:
>
> "I pray for you," says the Catholic.
> "Don't you dare," replies the atheist.

3.10 Invisible Religion

Or is there something like an "invisible religion", which manifests itself in fluid spirituality and nothing else but a "sense and taste for the infinite" (Friedrich Schleiermacher)?

The Austrian psychiatrist Victor Frankl writes in his book "The Unconscious God" about "the revealing unconscious religiosity of man". He calls this the "unknown and unconscious God", which every human being is supposed to carry within him, which needs to be made conscious. Perhaps this is exactly what the success of the dear God is connected with: namely, that one does not see him (for more on this see Chap. 6. A power, greater than ourselves: Conceptions of God).

3.11 Belief—what is it?

*"Belief means,
believing in something,
of which one knows,
that it is not true."*
(Mark Twain)

What is it actually—belief? The term belief has a religious and an everyday dimension. In everyday life, it hides the basic willingness to consider a certain fact as true, which we have not checked or could not check. Some speak of the "inner altar of certainty": belief is therefore certainty without evidence. For believers, no explanation is necessary. However—many do not even know exactly what they actually believe (or are supposed to believe).

When things go well, belief is integrated and synthesized worldview and thus helpful. It becomes problematic when belief as a lived introject in a person festers like a stake in the flesh and cannot be integrated because there is an identification with the aggressor in the personal life history that is difficult to resolve. Re***thinking*** is already difficult for many—"Re***believing***" (i.e., finding another belief) is even more difficult.

In addition: The transitions between knowledge, belief, religiosity, and gullibility are fluid: "Do you still believe—or do you already know?" is a slogan of the religion-critical Giordano Bruno Foundation (GBS). Undoubtedly, much is believed, but little is known. "Think instead of pray" is therefore the tenor of the GBS. But what can we—apart from banalities—really know? Therefore, a goal could be: to believe with a clear head. Belief reduces complexity, but I can think about it and reflect on my own position and justify it for myself: Religious simplicity can very well be linked with scientific diversity.

> **Heretical question** Do I rise in faith or do I sink in faith?

On the religious level, belief means that believers usually believe in a transcendent reality. In our cultural circle, this is often associated with a higher being (God, Allah, Yahweh), in other Far Eastern cultures it is associated with a belief in a rather impersonal energy (Tao, Chi, Brahman …).

3.12 "faith" and "believe"

The German word Glauben is translated into English with two very different terms. A distinction is made between "faith" and "believe".

Under **faith**, belief is understood in the sense of general trust in God as a supporting and shaping force of human existence. One could also say it is a kind of "primal trust", a kind of primal ground that is identical in all meaningful religions in all cultures at all times. If it is possible to penetrate to this point, religion can be healing.

> *"The love for an eternal and infinite thing*
> *nourishes the soul with the only real joy*
> *and is free of all sorrow."*
> *(Baruch Spinoza)*

In contrast to faith, **believe** refers to the concrete beliefs and doctrines of individual religions. These beliefs are highly influenced by culture and the zeitgeist at the time of their creation and are more or less meaningful. The beliefs between the different religions are very different and are the background of many religious conflicts and religious wars. Often these begin with the motto "Only we have the right faith and we must proselytize you. If necessary, with fire and sword. For if you are not willing, we need violence". In the worst case, this turns religions into terms of struggle.

> **Heretical Objection**
>
> The belief of the individual can gladly be his kingdom of heaven. After all, the world is big enough for everyone to be wrong in their own way.
>
> No one wants to take away his subjective view. It only becomes a problem when he elevates his subjective truth to the only, eternally valid religious truth and forces others to adopt this view. Otherwise, the threat is the torture chamber, the witch hammer, the stake—or at least social exclusion.

This side of belief is so resistant to arguments because they were usually adopted without scrutiny. If one were to think critically about it, the entire belief system could be shaken—and this could possibly be accompanied by a high degree of personal insecurity: One cannot know what one does not know.

*"So the course of a man's life is usually this,
that he is fooled by hope,
dances into the arms of death."
(Arthur Schopenhauer)*

That is why all religions always invoke the certainty of faith: "A mighty fortress is our God", is a line from a hymn attributed to Martin Luther.

> **Heretical Objection** Certainty of faith is the high art of graciously granted self-deception.

3.13 Nihilism

*"All religions are based on a mythical
more or less nonsensical basic idea."
(Frederick the Great)*

The professor of philosophy at the University of Münster, Werner Schneiders, who died in 2021, writes in his book "The Globalization of Nihilism" (Freiburg/Munich, 2019, Karl Alber Publishing House):

"Even religion is not a mighty fortress. Even in the unlikely event of a victory by any religion or even the united religions of this world, nihilism remains fundamentally intact, for it even dwells in the heart of religion. Every religion has so far carried the germ of decay within itself, doubt always gnaws at one's own faith. In short, nihilism is probably not to be eradicated by religion, at least not by any salto mortale" (p. 112 f.).

3.14 Serendipity

In New High German, it is called "Serendipity", wisdom and intelligent luck, when you stumble upon something you weren't even looking for, but which advances you in a surprising way.

*"I find everything related to religion interesting."
But it irritates me that otherwise intelligent people
take it so seriously."
(Douglas Adams, Hitchhiker's Guide to the Galaxy)*

The proportion of thinking people who can no longer adopt the traditional systems of meaning suffer from a kind of "metaphysical dissatisfaction". And it seems to be increasing. Anyone who cannot or does not want to adopt an off-the-shelf system of meaning (like those offered by religions) must assemble or cobble together their own system of meaning. This is still common in the esoteric scene: a bit of Buddhism from here, a pinch of Christianity, some shamanism and a lot of diffuse esotericism—from Bach flowers and astrology to gemstone therapy and Native American sweat lodges to trance dances and kinesiology. It is not uncommon to find the desires of the old mystics in this search: "It is the goal of all those endowed with intelligence to become God," Hermes Trismegistos announced many hundreds of years ago. But this search is not entirely safe: "Whoever climbs higher than he should, falls deeper than he wanted."

So if you don't want to get stuck in the esoteric swamp of belief, it's good to give room to doubt here too: "Distrust the idyll," said André Heller. Even if it's good to be able to trust: Don't switch off your mind.

> **Heretical Objection** There is hardly any field where there is as much fraud, self-deception and hypocrisy as in the field of religions.

Although no one knows God's plan—must, should, can we therefore believe? As the Cologne cabaret artist Jürgen Becker said: "Religion is when you die anyway."

References

Blume, R. G., Kropfberger, K.: Homo systemicus, Göttingen 2020 (Vandenhoeck und Ruprecht)
Bucher, Anton A.: Psychologie der Spiritualität, Weinheim 2007 (Beltz)
Blume, R. G., Kropfberger, K.: Homo systemicus, Göttingen 2020 (Vandenhoeck und Ruprecht)
Eco, Umberto, Martini, Carlo M.: Woran glaubt, wer nicht glaubt? Augsburg 2005 (Weltbild)
Frankl, Viktor E.: Der Wille zum Sinn – Bern 1972, 2. Auflage (Huber)
Gebser, Jean: Ursprung und Gegenwart, Köln 1949 (Novalis)
Hampten-Turner, Charles: Modelle des Menschen, Weinheim 1982 (Beltz)
Henningsen, Peter: Werkzeuge der Erkenntnis, Basel 1984 (Sphinx)
Holl, Hans Günter: Das lockere und das strenge Denken, Weinheim 1985 (Beltz)

Hellinger, Bert: Religion, Psychotherapie, Seelsorge, München 2000 (Kösel)
Huisman, Denis: Philosophie für Einsteiger, Reinbek 1983 (Rowohlt)
Huisman, Denis: Philosophie für Einsteiger, Reinbek 1983 (Rowohlt)
Janich, Peter: Was ist Erkenntnis? München 2000 (C.H. Beck)
Jaeger, Lars: Supermacht Wissenschaft, Gütersloh 2012 (Gütersloher Verlagshaus)
Jaeger, Lars: Wissenschaft und Spiritualität, Berlin/Heidelberg 2017 (Springer)
Jarzombek, Dieter (Hrsg.): Freiheit, die wir meinen, Berlin 2014 (Lit-Verlag Dr. W. Hopf)
Janich, Peter: Was ist Erkenntnis? München 2000 (C.H. Beck)
Küng, Hans: Existiert Gott? Freiburg 2017 (Herder)
Kolbe, Christoph: Heilung oder Hindernis – Religion bei Freud, Adler, Fromm, Jung und Frankl, Stuttgart 1986 (Kreuz)
Moser, Tilmann: Gott auf der Couch, Gütersloh 2011 (Gütersloher Verlagshaus)
Moser, Tilmann: Gottesvergiftung, Frankfurt 1976 (Suhrkamp)
Penrose, Roger: Das Große, das Kleine und der menschliche Geist, Heidelberg/Berlin 1998 (Spektrum)
Rensch, Bernhard: Das universelle Weltbild, Frankfurt 1977 (Fischer-TB)
Richter, Horst E.: Der Gotteskomplex, Gießen 2005 (Psychosozial)
Schweid, Richard: Sehnsucht nach Unsterblichkeit, Gütersloh 2008 (Gütersloher Verlagshaus)
Schneiders, Werner: Die Globalisierung des Nihilismus, Freiburg/München, 2019 (Verlag Karl Alber)
Wittgenstein, Ludwig: Philosophische Untersuchungen, Frankfurt 1971 (Suhrkamp)

Left

Buddhismus: Kernaussagen – Religion – Kultur – Planet Wissen (planet-wissen.de) (Stand: 18.9.2023)
Serendipität – Wikipedia (Stand: 18.9.2023)

4

The Smaller (or More Confused) the Mind, the More Concrete must be the Image of God and Certainty

> **Summary**
>
> This chapter deals with the various attitudes and basic beliefs about faith and how religion affects the individual. It discusses the benefits believers derive from their faith, through which they gain orientation, guidelines, and support, but also where they feel constrained and patronized by religion and, in the worst case, develop "religious neuroses". A typology of believers is presented—from credulous and reflective to compulsively anxious and dogmatically know-it-all to church haters or skeptics and agnostics. Then you will find a small faith test (focus on Christianity) in the chapter.

4.1 Do You Really know What You Believe (or should Believe)?

Many people believe they know what they believe. In reality, many beliefs are rather unconscious and they are not clear about what they actually believe or should believe. Many, for example, call themselves Christians and only have a vague idea of what Christianity actually entails. Therefore, here is a small faith test:

4.2 Small Faith Test (Focus on Christianity)

- Do you believe that God exists? If yes—what do you think about him and what can you say about him?

- What is God for you (e.g.: "God is a personal unity", "God is an impersonal energy", "God is in everything", "God does not exist for me" …)?
- If there is a God for you—is there also an adversary of God for you (personal: Satan, Devil, Lucifer or the evil/bad)?
- Is Jesus Christ God incarnate for you—and at all a God?
- Do you believe that Jesus died for us through his atonement?
- Do you believe in the "Immaculate Conception" of Mary (virgin birth), through which Jesus is said to have come into the world, as Jesus was conceived by the Holy Spirit?
- Do you believe in the resurrection of Jesus after his death?
- Do you believe in the (bodily) ascension of Christ (and/or) Mary?
- What is the Trinity (God the Father—Son—Holy Spirit) for you?
- For Catholics: Is the Pope God's representative on earth for you?
- Do you consider him infallible when he speaks "ex cathedra"?
- Do you consider the Bible (or the Quran, the Torah, the Bhagavad Gita …) a holy book? On what grounds?
- Do other realities exist for you? What do they look like and how did they come about?
- What happens from your point of view after death—for you and with you?
- Do you believe in the Last Judgment or reincarnation—or what?
- If we resurrect bodily after the Last Judgment—in which body do we do that? As a 6-year-old, when you still believed every nonsense? As an 18-year-old, when you didn't believe anything anymore? Or as a 58-year-old, when you started believing again?
- Do you believe in "eternal life" (after death)?
- Do you believe in heaven and hell? What do they look like?
- Symbolization ability: Is there something that is holy for you? What is it—and why is it holy for you?
- What other questions do you have about your religion?

4.3 Don't believe Everything you think: Religious Neuroses

The personal attitude towards one's own faith can greatly shape the general attitude towards life: How I believe and what religion means to me and my life is highly individual. Whether I feel safe, accepted, and welcomed in this world largely depends on what I have learned throughout my own life story. If I experienced a religious perspective as helpful and supportive in childhood, it can be a blessing to be able to believe. Whether I need a—however shaped—image of God and religious belief system for this is very different from person to person. Some people do not need religious support and guidelines for this kind of basic trust.

It is quite different if I have experienced religious rules and duties as incomprehensible introjects ("like a stake in the flesh") with non-integrable commandments and prohibitions. Perhaps they have always remained foreign to the core of my personality, or I have even vehemently resisted them because of the patronization and confinement. If this inner conflict lasts long enough and is intense enough, even "religious neuroses" can develop.

The benefits believers gain from their faith, through which they receive orientation, guidelines, and support, depend exactly on such conditions. Therefore, it is definitely helpful to have a certain reflective distance from one's own belief system: Don't believe everything you think.

> **Heresy Interjection** I think that one can and may imagine all sorts of nonsense. One can also develop all sorts of theories about it. However, they should be able to withstand a reality test. That is, they must not contradict the proven findings of the sciences.

4.4 Holy Simplicity or Religious Diversity?

When you look at how many very different religions and faiths there are in the world, you might ask yourself: Why did I end up in this belief system? Does it have to do with where—in which culture and in which social class—I grew up? Did I choose my faith freely? Does it actually suit me? Do I feel comfortable in it? What keeps and binds me to this faith today?

> **For Reflection** But why do we always end up with religions? Why are we actually looking for a system of meaning? What do we want and what do we actually need it for?

4.5 Typology of Believers and Their Attitude Towards Faith

This section introduces various groups of people who I have encountered in my over 40 years of work with people in therapy, counseling, supervision, and seminars, who have different attitudes towards faith and religion. These are experiences that I have encountered in my professional life as a psychologist and psychotherapist and that I have summarized in certain clusters.

4.5.1 Gullible: "Unreflective-naive folk religion"

The gullible person usually absorbed religion with their mother's milk. He (or she) grew up in a more or less religious household. The family, father and mother, siblings were and are rooted in religion—possibly over many generations. The family regularly attended church services and individual family members often engaged in the church community. Just like a fish that doesn't think about what water is, the gullible person has no critical distance to their religion. He/she is baptized and has gone through various religious initiations: communion, confirmation, confirmation, church wedding, etc. The image of God is consistently positive. The faith is a kind of childlike faith, often associated with goodnight prayers, guardian angels, and a deep trust in God and the world: Everything is and will be good. For the gullible, no explanation is necessary. For them, their perspective is the only possible one and they do not understand that others could see it very differently.

4.5.2 Reflective believers: "Consciously and justifiably religious"

Reflective believers have already thought about religion and the meaning of religiosity. The perspective is reflective and at least partly justified. He/she may have already gone through various (faith) crises but has always returned to their own religion and does not really question it. God is always just a prayer away for him/her. He/she can (usually) perceive that there are other people with different faith principles.

4.5.3 Dogmatic know-it-alls: "You know it—but I know it better"

The dogmatic know-it-all is overly convinced of his religion. He believes that his perspective is the only correct one. He/she has pronounced missionary ambitions and tries to convince everyone else of his/her point of view. Dogmatic know-it-alls can be found not only in so-called sects, but also on the fringes of traditional major churches. The background is often the hidden (and more or less conscious) fear that their own perspective might not be correct. Therefore, he is only allowed to think about his religion within the given boundaries. His attitude is best characterized by the following sentence: "Jesus is the answer—what was the question again?" Often he has been indoctrinated with religion (sometimes since his childhood), in the worst case he has been "drilled" into the religious perspective. He/she cannot (and does not want to) detach himself/herself from the dogmatic perspective because he/she considers it to be the only true and correct one.

4.5.4 Compulsive Fear believers: "Tormented by a guilty conscience"

For the compulsive fear believer, the fear of breaking rules is paramount. He/she fears that if he/she does not follow the rules, something terrible will happen. Here, the separation between good and evil, black and white is very clear. If he (in the Christian area) does not follow the commandments of God proclaimed by the pastor or in the Bible, then he feels that he is damned to hell and the devil gains power over him. The transitions to the dogmatic know-it-all can be fluid.

4.5.5 Skeptics, Rationalists, Scientists, Atheists, Naturalists: "I can't comment on that"

Skeptics can present many reasons for their skepticism. If they are scientifically oriented, they find no evidence that there could be a God, therefore religion is considered nonsense: "Do you still believe or do you already know?" is often the motto. "Freedom of religion instead of being without religion" is usually the rational or scientific basic attitude. As a naturalist, he/she may have a romantic connection to "Mother Earth". Sometimes in this group you also find those who would like to believe if they could only believe.

4.5.6 Cynics: "Ironical Attitude"

Cynics are characterized by an ironic attitude towards religion. They make no statements about whether there is a higher power. They often consider religion to be nonsense, God or gods do not exist for them. The transitions to the skeptic and church hater can sometimes be fluid.

4.5.7 Religion and Church Haters: "Abolish the Churches!"

Religion and church haters only see the negative sides of what religion has caused in the past centuries: from witch burning to religious wars and psychological disfigurements to the abuse cases of the last decades in the churches. They like to use the term "religiots" for church believers.

4.5.8 Superficial: "I'm not Interested in Questions of Meaning—I don't care about religion"

Superficial people do not think about whether there is a God at all. Questions of meaning are far away for them. They are indifferent to religion and religious organizations. They live for the day and the main focus is on fun and pleasure. Kurt von Vigier put it this way: "The pious live healthier, but the sinner lives more beautifully." Only in crises does the question of meaning become a topic for them at all. This is probably the largest group of the Central European population.

4.5.9 Agnostics: What can we really know?

Agnostics are primarily questioners. They do not dare to make statements about whether there is a God or any other kind of higher power. They are seekers and are not satisfied with hasty off-the-shelf answers. Although agnostics may not believe in God, their motto is best expressed in the Jewish sentence: "You are closer to God when you ask a question than when you give an answer." Today's truth can be untrue for them tomorrow. They often care about the mystery of life and its religious embellishment.

Certainly, this typology is crude and there are a multitude of transitions between the individual groups of people and various mixed types. The typology presented is not the result of statistically valid and reliable tests, but (as already mentioned above) is the result of experiences with people who I have encountered in psychotherapies, coachings or seminars and whom I have tried to systematically capture. It would certainly be interesting if the results could be statistically verified within the framework of a research project.

4.6 Fit: Who ends up in which Religious Group?

Certainly, these subgroups cannot be cleanly separated from each other. There are transitions and commonalities between these groups of people. Since the process is very individual and highly complex, it is worth looking very closely at each individual person. In which religious group does he/she end up? Where does he/she stay? In which religion does he/she feel at home or rooted—and/or is bound by which methods? (Answers to this see: 14.7 Fit: How religion and faith become a problematic cult).

References

Alexander, Pat und David: Das große Handbuch zur Bibel, Witten 2001 (SCM-Brockhaus)
Bork, Uwe: Kleines Lexikon biblischer Irrtümer, Gütersloh 2009 (Gütersloher Verlagshaus)
Bernhardt, Reinhold: Der Absolutheitsanspruch des Christentums, Gütersloh 1990 (Gütersloher Verlagshaus)
Ciupka-Schön, B., Becks, H.: Himmel und Hölle – Religiöse Zwänge erkennen und bewältigen, Ostfildern 2018 (Patmos)
Frankl, Viktor E.: Der Wille zum Sinn – Bern 1972, 2nd edn, (Huber)
Ferrucci, Franco: Die Schöpfung – Das Leben Gottes, von ihm selbst erzählt, Frankfurt 1990 (Fischer-TB)
Koch, K. et al. (Eds.): Reclams Bibellexikon, Stuttgart 1992 (Reclam)
Kunter, Katharina: 500 Jahre Protestantismus, Gütersloh 2011, (Gütersloher Verlagshaus)
Metz, Wulf (Hrsg): Handbuch Weltreligionen, Wuppertal 2003, 5th edn. (Brockhaus)
Mears, Henrietta: Alles was man über die Bibel wissen muss, Wuppertal 2004 (Brockhaus)
Ruffing, Reiner: Kleines Lexikon wissenschaftlicher Irrtümer, Gütersloh 2011 (Gütersloher Verlagshaus)
Smith, Huston: Eine Wahrheit, viele Wege – Die großen Religionen der Welt, Freiburg 1993 (Bauer)
Satinover, Jeffrey: Die verborgene Botschaft der Bibel, München 1997 (Goldmann)
Schmelzer, Carsten St.: Heilung – Was wir glauben und erwarten dürfen, Witten 2013 (SCM-Brockhaus)

Part II

How Religions Became What They Are

5

The Past Gods: How Religions Originated—and where They have Evolved: From the Stone Age to Today

> **Summary**
>
> This chapter deals with the emergence of religions from the earliest beginnings in the Stone Age, when natural events were associated with personalized gods, through the first cultural developments with increasingly differentiated images of gods, to the opulent world of gods of ancient India with its many hundred gods, who mostly embodied certain characteristics and had very human traits—similar to ancient Egypt and also in the Pantheon, the heaven of gods of the ancient Greeks and Romans. In addition, this chapter presents the development of religions from polytheism to monotheistic religions: Judaism, Christianity, and Islam.

"God sleeps in the stones,
breathes in the plants,
dreams in the animals
and awakens in humans."
(spiritual wisdom)

In the past, the vegetative soul of plants was distinguished from the animal soul of animals and the human soul, which was considered immortal and had a connection to the world soul (spirit, Ruach, Pneuma), which subtly permeated the entire cosmos.

5.1 Where did the Gods come from?

In the course of human evolutionary history, all societies have developed concepts of God and religious systems. Is man therefore something like a "Homo religiosus" who needs religion as a system of meaning?

But: How did people actually come to invent God and gods? Every people needs and has its legends and narratives, which also reflect the creation myths of folk religions. These were passed on orally for many generations and later written down at some point, which often exposed them to the danger of becoming unquestionable dogma. The further religions developed, the more a kind of "omnipotence delusion" developed among their members: The religious leaders believed that their religion was the only correct one and would apply for all times into eternity. Until the next religion comes up … But let's start at the very beginning.

5.2 From the Big Bang to the Emergence of Hominids

The Big Bang happened about 14.8 billion years ago. It then took about 10 billion years for our Earth to emerge from the matter whirling around in space (so about 4.4 billion years ago). It also took many hundreds of millions of years for the boiling chaos to eventually become the somewhat solid Earth's core.

We are talking here about dimensions of time that strain and sometimes exceed our imagination: Who can really imagine and empathize with what millions or even billions of years really means—where we nowadays rather think in seconds, minutes, hours, days, and years?

Because the further path from inanimate matter via single cells, plants and animals—to the precursors of humans also seems almost endless. It also takes many millions of years from then on until the emergence of humans in the course of evolution…

If we go back in human evolutionary history, one can of course ask: When does being human actually begin? Even if the transition was certainly fluid and took place on many levels: Until when were we primarily animal and when did we become human?

> **Excursion: Transition from animal to human—can animals (religiously) believe?**
> Surely animals can develop something like (primordial) trust. But does this have anything to do with what we humans call religion? At least probably not in our sense. Because for that, it would probably need a different brain structure, dealing with future and past and questions of meaning, the ability to develop and symbolize fantasies. Religion is linguistic—animals think, but certainly not linguistically.

But when did it all start?

It is about 8 million years ago that the evolutionary line of humans split off from that of the great apes. With Australopithecus, a first hominid genus emerged 4 million years ago (brain volume—still like that of chimpanzees—approx. 400 cubic centimeters, strong molars, only predominantly bipedal locomotion).

5.3 Genus Homo

The oldest precursors of the genus Homo in the narrower sense (2.5–1.5 million years ago) are considered to be **Homo rudolfensis** and **Homo habilis** (brain size: approx. 700 cubic centimeters). They were already able to use and manufacture the first stone tools, which required anticipatory planning for later use. They also gradually managed to tame fire.

Homo erectus made a significant developmental leap about 2 million years ago: His brain had a volume of 1200 cubic centimeters, and his body skeleton and size were almost equivalent to those of modern humans. These ancestors of ours must have developed something like the beginnings of a language, as tool production was more complex and could no longer be achieved through mere imitation.

Between 700,000 and 300,000 years ago, **Homo heidelbergensis** lived. His classification in the human family tree is disputed. His brain volume is between 1,200 and 1,400 cubic centimeters, his body size is 1.60–1.70 m, and he weighs between 50 and 60 kg. He could make stone tools and wooden spears. These were signs that he could hunt larger animals, usually in small groups.

But when did something like the precursors of religions develop—and what did it depend on? Throughout evolutionary history, the brain of the genus Homo grew larger, the gait became more upright, the resemblance to apes disappeared more and more, manual dexterity improved, and the first forms of linguistic communication developed.

5.4 Neanderthals and Homo Sapiens

Although the genus Homo sapiens is spoken of from the period of 300,000 BC, the Neanderthals lived about 120,000 to 27,000 years ago—thus a parallel development. And it still took a while for our ancestors to come up with something like the first images of gods.

In the very early times, when people still roamed the earth as hunting and gathering nomadic hordes—always following the prey animals—little is known about their conceptions of gods. However, uncontrollable natural phenomena (volcanic eruptions, thunderstorms, storm surges, wild animals …) probably caused fears, dread, and feelings of helplessness in the Stone Age people, which they tried to banish through personalization.

Even gentler natural cycles, such as the interplay of the seasons, lead to the emergence of ideas, inner images of oversized powers (higher beings, gods, spirits, devils, angels …). Some of these powers are experienced as good and benevolent, others as malicious and dangerous. And there develops in the groups of Stone Age people the desire for appeasement, comprehensibility, and connection with these higher forces. Thus, the first myths, beliefs, cults, and (sacrificial) rituals emerge—usually associated with feelings of hope, redemption, protection, and connection.

5.5 Belief in the Stone Age

Imagine sitting in a Stone Age cave with your tribe in winter. Outside, a fierce storm is brewing and a bitterly cold winter wind is swirling the snowflakes. You are somewhat protected in the cave. A campfire flickers in front of you and you try to warm yourself by the fire. You have—as was usual in the Stone Age—no ideas or knowledge about weather phenomena, but sit more or less frightened and shocked like the other clan members in front of the fire. You huddle together and into your bear skin because of these overpowering forces. The shadows flicker on the wall. You feel at the mercy of these external powers and inner fantasies and frightening images rise within you. The uncertainty is great—also because someone from the clan has just died. Conversations are so far only monosyllabic and limited …

5.6 Origins of Consciousness

In contrast to animals, the then Homo sapiens developed beginnings of what is now called consciousness—even if it was perhaps only rudimentary in the Stone Age. Homo sapiens consciously or unconsciously experiences that his self is separate from the environment. He gradually begins to think in causal relationships. Even though the Stone Age people probably still lived more instinctively and the most important thing was to survive the next few days, they primarily perceived the world through their sensory organs (seeing, hearing, touching, smelling, tasting) and stored it in memory. A gradual decoupling of need and satisfaction develops. Gradually, short-term satisfaction is sacrificed for a longer-term goal (also due to group pressure). Something like impulse control and frustration tolerance emerge. Due to the conformity pressure of the small group, common norms emerge that prescribe group-specific rules: This is right and that is wrong. For each individual, it is the (more or less conscious) task to sort and evaluate these experiences in order to survive as an individual and in the group. Gradually, the ability develops to form lasting internal representations of what happens, to be able to remember it and to link it with previous experiences in order to draw the right conclusions and develop the appropriate actions.

Because already from the Stone Age, our ancestors had to have something like a sense of time and develop goal-oriented ideas of the future—to be able to form hypotheses—and to believe in something. E.g. what or who might have caused this winter storm and what can be done to appease these (imagined) entities. Perhaps these powers, later called gods, can be appeased by sacrifices? But also the question of what happens to the deceased who now lies lifeless here, and where the living part of him might have gone?

The German-Swiss philosopher Jean Gebser (1905–1973) spent a long time dealing with the individual-psychological development of humans and formulated five structural stages of human consciousness development (Jean Gebser, Origin and Present, 1949):

- Archaic
- Magical
- Mythical
- Mental
- Integral

These five stages were later revised by the American consciousness researcher Ken Wilber from around 1975 and presented in a modified form in his books.

5.7 Burial Rituals

Already around 100,000 BC, there were probably simple burial rituals and a belief in an existence beyond death (possibly through "soul migration") developed. Perhaps it is primarily the inability to understand what death is, and the question of what might happen after death, that evoke this horror. This may have been the cause for the Stone Age people trying to banish this uncertainty with first religious rituals.

So it was probably the Neanderthals who from 60,000 BC as the first hominid group did not simply leave their dead (unlike the animals), but buried them in ceremonial burials with proper burial rites.

5.8 Grave Goods

At some point, the custom also arose to give the dead grave goods for their last journey. At first, these were only small figures, food or simple tools. In the Neolithic Age (from 10,000 BC), the grave goods—especially for the clan leaders—became more opulent: jewelry, ceramic objects, weapons were probably intended to help them survive in the "other world".

What can be said from this: If a deceased person is given objects to take into the grave, this is an indication that this community believes in a (continued) life after death. Especially since these are often objects that the deceased could have needed to continue living in another world.

5.9 Pre-religious Forms of Belief

The American consciousness psychologist and cult author Ken Wilber writes in his book "Halfway through Evolution" that early humans were not only hunters and gatherers, but also "magicians".

From 30,000 BC, spiritual rituals with specific symbols and signs developed—probably also independently of burials. Because Stone Age people had developed initial abilities for symbolization. Thus, a regular ancestor cult (Manism) developed among various tribes, in which deceased ancestors were honored. For the animistic ancestral figures were considered creators or helpers of certain phenomena (finding the right settlement place, influencing the weather, hunting luck, etc.)—or at least had an influence on them. These cultic rituals were probably often associated with drink, food, or fire sacrifices. It is likely that intense emotions were also mobilized communally (ecstasy, dances, trance, orgies), which also served to hold the group together.

What must not be forgotten: In the Stone Age, our ancestors died very early. The average life expectancy at that time was between 20 and 25 years. Many children died in the first four years of life. The reasons were diseases, lack of hygiene, poor nutrition, and everyday stresses.

5.10 Animism, Totemism, Shamanism

Pre-religious forms of belief in prehistoric times include animism, totemism, and shamanism.

Animism means that both living beings and inanimate objects would have a soul. This is also referred to as "all-soulness". According to this, the whole world is "ensouled" and it is about communicating with the souls of the whole world.

Totemism is the belief in the supernatural power of a totem. A totem is an animal, plant, or inanimate being that was later used and revered by clans as a tribal sign. It was magically and emotionally charged (or even sacred) and often symbolically stood for an (original) ancestor or relative of a people or clan.

Shamanism is the term for beliefs and spiritual practices practiced by shamans. Shamans were already important—sometimes even sacred—people in prehistoric times, especially in tribal cultures. A shaman (man or woman) was already a spiritual leader among many indigenous peoples. For these women and men from the clan, who understood how to heal with herbs and other aids, were already considered particularly important people (shamans), as they were often (as in later tribal cultures) attributed the above-mentioned abilities to have a direct line to the supernatural world of spirits and gods. They saw themselves as mediators ("medium") between the sensual-physical and the supernatural-spiritual world and wanted to be their mouthpiece. Many shamans already claimed at that time to possess and/or channel supernatural powers and to be able to heal diseases. Shamanism is considered the oldest verifiable form of (pre-)religious thinking. Shamanism has been verifiable since the Upper Paleolithic (about 30,000 years ago).

"Nature is the hidden God."
(Friedrich W. J. Schelling,
German philosopher, 1775–1854)

5.11 Belief in the Supernatural: Spirits and Gods

Stone Age people probably believed in spirits or gods, which they tried to capture on rock paintings and/or appease.

In addition, many of the found female figurines could represent (fertility) goddesses. And there are indications that there were regular sacrifices to appease the supernatural powers. The gods of that time were nature gods—similar to later among the Germans, where Thor was the god of thunder and lightning, Frigg, the protective goddess of motherhood, or Tyr the god of war.

5.12 Cave Paintings

Stone Age people were surprisingly creative artists. They painted both individual animals and hunting scenes as well as supernatural beings and fleeing herds of animals on the cave walls. More than 300 sites of cave paintings are now known worldwide.

The oldest rock paintings were recently found in Indonesia and are 45,500 years old (a life-size wild boar). The most well-known in our latitudes are the paintings in the French cave of Lascaux from the Neolithic period (about 20,000 BC), the Chauvet cave (36,000 BC), and the Spanish Altamira cave (14,000 BC).

Painting was probably related to cults and rites. For the images may have served as a symbolic language to record hunting techniques and migration routes. According to the ideas of the time, the souls of the depicted beings are probably preserved in the rock paintings, which could be brought back to life by painting, by touching the images, but also by performing cultic rituals.

5.13 Sedentism

A stone monument on the Turkish mountain Göbekli Tepe, (circa 11,500 BC) probably indicates a complex death cult. Göbekli Tepe is one of the oldest structures of mankind worldwide. They were created at a time when hunters and gatherers became sedentary farmers. This building is considered one of the oldest temple complexes in the world, where offerings were made to gods.

The concrete and later fixed ideas of gods probably only emerged when our ancestors began to settle down about 10,000 years ago, practicing agriculture, fishing, and livestock farming, and building fences around their properties and protective walls around their settlements. These settlements initially consisted of huts, tent camps, caves, and rock shelters. However, the larger the individual settlements became and the more people lived in them, the more they developed into proper villages that had to develop an infrastructure, e.g., fortifications of the buildings, irrigation systems, etc.

This also led to the division of labor: precursors of professions emerged (farmer, potter, carpenter, blacksmith, medicine man…). And this also made it possible for a part of the settlers to engage in religion and art (e.g., shamans).

Only from then on did a more stable role distribution in the clan and a lasting hierarchy develop, in which the differences between the individual people and clans were more or less concretely defined. Thus, as the communities grew larger, increasingly stark differences between rich and poor, between masters, servants, and slaves developed. This played a particularly important role in the early cities.

5.14 Emergence of Cities

Gradually, the first early civilizations emerged: Mesopotamia, Asia Minor, Crete, Egypt, India, China—also in South and Central America. These developed mainly in the cities.

According to recent archaeological findings, there were already around 3000 BC worldwide 15 cities and city-like settlements. By 1500 BC, there were already over 100 cities worldwide. And already 67 million people lived on earth.

Jericho (in Palestine) is probably the oldest city in the world that was continuously inhabited. It was founded around 10,000 BC. Thus, Jericho has outpaced the two cities of Eridu and Uruk located in the Mesopotamian land between the Euphrates and Tigris, which were long considered the oldest cities in the world and were founded around 5000 BC. Archaeological research has also shown that other cities like the Turkish Catalhöyük (7500 BC) and the Bulgarian Plovdiv (around 6000 BC) were older than the Mesopotamian cities.

Urbanity created a new situation in which people lived together in a confined space and had to get along with the existing infrastructure. Thus, the gods also changed and new (pre-)forms of religion developed.

5.15 Mesopotamia

Mesopotamia refers to an area between the Euphrates and Tigris and is therefore also called the land of two rivers. It lies between Iraq, Syria, and Anatolia. Here the first high cultures were founded. It is the home of the Sumerians, who immigrated to Mesopotamia around the 5th millennium BC.

The early cities in Mesopotamia show that people had already thought about and planned for the future of the city at a very early stage, and there was long-term planning from the time of foundation: The city was oriented according to the main wind directions. There was a regular, walled, step-like temple district ("Zikkurat") which was laid out at right angles, and the city walls and canals were fortified and stable.

The Sumerian religion is considered the first religion that can be recorded in writing. It inspired later cultures such as the Akkadians, Assyrians, and Babylonians. The Sumerian gods are (alongside the Egyptian ones) among the oldest gods we know by name. Because even if there were gods in earlier times, they did not bear lasting names—at least none that were handed down. Because the archaic gods were simply equated with natural forces: heaven and earth, sun and moon, order and chaos…

The earliest centers of the Sumerians in the 5th and 4th millennium BC are the cities of Eridu and Uruk. The most important deity is "Enki" ("Lord of the Earth"). But the Sumerians believed in many different deities. In addition to "Enki", the main deities were "An" and "Enlil". But in principle, there was a god or goddess for every natural phenomenon (Tiamat, Inanna, Utu, Ereshkigal…). As a result, each Sumerian city worshiped its own patron god. The priests were not only spiritual leaders and servants of God, but they also administered the city as secular leaders. Around 2750 BC, Gilgamesh, the legendary king of Uruk in Mesopotamia, ruled.

5.16 Ancient Egypt

The oldest cities in Egypt were Memphis, Achmim, and Thebes. Each of these cities had its own city god. In Thebes, it was Ptah, the patron saint of craftsmen. In Achmim, the local god was Min, who had a close connection to Horus, the sky god. Thebes, which was located in Upper Egypt very close to today's Luxor, had Amun as its city god, the god of wind and fertility.

The Egyptians, who will remain in the world's memory primarily for their pyramids, already had a proper and differentiated pantheon with well over 20 main gods and many minor gods. Since the Egyptians had developed a differentiated sign and script language (hieroglyphics) and many Westerners have since visited the country as tourists, many of the Egyptian gods are already known:

- Atum—the creator god
- Hathor—the goddess of love and beauty
- Aton—the sun god
- Horus—the sky god
- Anubis—the god with the jackal head
- Bastet—the goddess with the cat head
- Isis—the mother and protective deity
- Osiris—the god of the dead
- Nut—the goddess who swallows the sun at night and gives birth to it again in the morning
- Sobek—the crocodile god
- Etc.

All these deities represent certain themes and fields of activity and have designated characteristics. Sometimes they are benevolent towards humans and help, sometimes they are dangerous or even malicious.

Pharaohs, as rulers of the country, were something like (semi-)gods on earth, who were supposed to lead and guide the people. They issued a multitude of religious and civil laws in the long history of ancient Egypt.

The term ancient Egypt refers to the period from about 3000 BC to 395 AD.

This long period of ancient Egypt is (repeatedly interrupted by so-called intermediate periods) divided into three kingdoms:

- The Old Kingdom (2707–2216 BC) is also called the "Pyramid Age" because the first and most important pyramids were built during this time (Great Pyramid of Giza, around 2500 BC).
- In the Middle Kingdom (2137–1781 BC), the Egyptian central state gradually disintegrated. Therefore, the relocation of the capital from Memphis to Thebes was of central importance and there were several internal power struggles for the pharaoh's throne.

- New Kingdom (1550–1070 BC): Egypt had a new golden age at the beginning of this era. The pharaohs pursued a large-scale expansion policy and Egypt experienced its greatest expansion. Around 1570 BC, the "Egyptian Book of the Dead" was created, which described the ideas of life after death. The division of the two main cities was also important: Thebes became the religious capital, Memphis the military capital.

The various transitional and intermediate periods in the long Egyptian history were characterized by many societal turbulences, political unrest, and power struggles.

5.17 Akhenaten

In relation to the Egyptian religion, something very important happened in 1356 BC. Amenophis IV initiated a complete change in the Egyptian worldview in a short time. To reduce the influence of the priesthood, all cults of gods were first banned and abolished. In his view, there was only one god (Aton, sun god). He henceforth called himself **Akhenaten** and had all temples dedicated to other gods repurposed or destroyed. During his reign, he moved to the new capital he founded, Akhet-Aton, which was located almost exactly in the middle between Memphis and Thebes. He thus completely turned away from **polytheism** and propagated—probably for the first time in human history—a strict **monotheism.** Thesis: There is only one god.

After Akhenaten died almost twenty years later, in 1336 BC, the subsequent pharaohs tried to return to the previous polytheistic worldview. The hatred of the priests, who had been disempowered by him, towards Akhenaten was so great that all images of him and his god Aton were subsequently destroyed to erase all memories of him. His son Tutankhamun, whose gilded death mask has made him famous to this day, was particularly prominent in this.

After the end of the New Kingdom, Egypt once again slid into a chaotic interlude and came under foreign rule (Assyrians, Alexander the Great, Romans). Cleopatra was the last (female) pharaoh. She had allied herself with Julius Caesar and the Roman Empire. From then on, Egypt remained a Roman province until the division of the Roman Empire in 395 AD.

5.18 Early India

There are a multitude of ancient writings that provide clues to the Hindu culture (and its predecessors) in India.

The Vedas are sacred texts, songs, hymns, and ritual instructions that were also passed down orally by old teachers over many generations in Sanskrit. There are four Vedas: Rigveda, Samaveda, and the white and black Yajurveda. There is evidence that the Rigveda Samhita originated in northwestern India between 1500 and 1200 BC.

The Upanishads are a collection of texts dating from the 5th and 4th centuries BC. They consist of a total of 108 writings.

The Bhagavad Gita is also one of the central scriptures of Hinduism. It was created between the 5th and 2nd centuries BC. It is a kind of spiritual poem that depicts a dialogue between Krishna, the earthly manifestation of the god Vishnu, and Arjuna, his student. It is about right action and duty to oneself.

Hinduism is a large polytheistic religion. There are several thousand Hindu gods. The most famous are:

- Brahma = Creator,
- Vishnu = Preserver,
- Shiva = the Destroyer.

Together, these three are known as the "Trimurti", the trinity of the divine. In addition, there are many other well-known Hindu deities: Rama, Krishna, Lakshmi, Saraswati, Hanuman (monkey god), Ganesha (elephant god) etc. (for more, see link: The most important goddesses and gods in Hinduism (yogaeasy.de) (as of: 18.09.2023).

5.19 The Heavenly Abode of the Olympians: Greek Gods

A similarly differentiated pantheon of gods as found among the Egyptians can also be found in ancient Greece. For the religion of the ancient Greeks was also polytheistic, and there was a large number of gods, which were hierarchically ordered. According to the myth, the highest 12 main gods lived in Olympus, the heavenly abode of the gods. There are highly complex narratives and many legends about this. For early on, the ancient Greeks saw in their gods anthropomorphic images of humans. The gods had good and bad characteristics, sometimes they were reflective and wise, sometimes they were moody, deceitful or even malicious. Many of the god figures probably arose through the merging of the religious ideas of the Aegean indigenous population with those of Indo-European and perhaps even Egyptian immigrants, which had begun around 2000 BC. However, it was primarily the poems of Homer and Hesiod, which around 800–700 BC significantly shaped the myth of the Greek heavenly abode of the gods. Here are the 12 main gods of Olympus:

- Zeus: Ruler of the Olympian gods, guardian of law and order
- His wife Hera: Goddess of marriage and childbirth, queen of heaven
- Demeter: Earth and fertility goddess
- Athena: Goddess of wisdom
- Dionysus: Fertility god and god of intoxication
- Hermes: Messenger of the gods, patron of merchants, travelers and thieves
- Aphrodite: Goddess of love and beauty
- Apollo: God of youth and prophecies
- Artemis: Goddess of hunting, goddess of childbirth
- Hephaestus: God of fire and blacksmithing
- Poseidon: God of the sea and earthquakes
- Ares: God of war

In addition, there were also a whole range of additional deities: e.g. Asclepius (healing god), Dike (goddess of justice), Eos (goddess of dawn), Eros (god of love), Hypnos (god of sleep) etc. There were also several local religions.

However, in ancient Greece, religion was increasingly expanded by philosophy. From around 600 BC, there was a veritable philosophical awakening, which was called the "Ionian Enlightenment". The philosophy of the pre-Socratics emerged: Thales, Anaximander and Anaximenes were the first representatives who also critically dealt with religion. Later, the philosopher and mathematician Pythagoras, born in 581 BC, was added. Parmenides (520–455 BC), Anaxagoras (499–428 BC), Socrates (469–399 BC) and later Plato (428–348 BC) and Aristotle (384–322 BC) took a completely different view of religions. The later philosophical schools of the Epicureans and the Stoics also dealt with questions of meaning. And especially the Stoics, founded around 300 BC by Zeno, had a strong influence—not only in Greece, but also later in Rome. Thus, the later Roman Emperor Marcus

Aurelius and the politician and philosopher Seneca were influenced by the Stoics.

5.20 Roman Gods

The Romans, like the Greeks, had an extensive pantheon of gods. Not only that—they "imported" a significant part of their gods from the Greek Olympus and simply relabeled them:

- Zeus became Jupiter
- Hera mutated into Juno
- Ares became Mars
- Aphrodite became Venus
- Poseidon became Neptune
- Athena was named Minerva
- And with Apollo, the god of light, they even kept the name entirely

The equating of foreign gods with their own became a characteristic of the Roman approach to foreign cultures.

However, the Roman pantheon included not only gods, but also demigods and other spiritual beings. Important in Roman religion was also that cult practices, rituals, and ceremonies played a significant role, in which the sacrifice of animals, plants, and other objects played an important part—and also interpretations, predictions, and prophecies of the priests were significant.

It is also important to know that the Roman religion—unlike the Greek one—was a state religion, i.e., a binding belief system. This also explains why there were later several persecutions of Christians (see Sect. 5.21). The Roman priesthood was hierarchically organized. At the top was the "Rex Sacrorum", then came the sacred officials ("Pontifices"), including the "Flamines" (sacrificial priests) and the "Vestalines" (priestesses of the goddess Vesta), who together performed the cult practices. All expressions of Roman mythology.

> **Excursus**
>
> What is a myth?
> A myth is a philosophical-religious narrative about the origin of the world, the cosmos, humans, God, and gods. The term is derived from the ancient

Greek word for narrative, legend. Originally, myths were passed on orally until the emergence of written language. The oldest written myth is the Epic of Gilgamesh.

Different types of myths can be distinguished:

- Cosmological myths deal with the origin of the world
- Theological M. describe the world of gods
- Anthropological M. explain the origin of humans
- Eschatological M. deal with the end of the world
- Etc.

People interpret the world and their own lives through myths in symbolic stories. Myths are explanatory patterns and often refer to fundamental and existential questions (meaning of life, life after death, good and evil …) and are therefore highly emotionally charged. Because myths have the psychological and social sense of making inexplicable processes explainable, and are therefore considered meaningful. If many myths belong together, one speaks of a mythology. Some people therefore refer to religions as mythologies and/or narratives.

5.21 Christianity: Beginnings and Important Events

No one knows what Jesus Christ really looked like, and yet an infinite number of images of him circulate. Jesus did not write any scriptures himself and all reports about him come from second or third hand. The story of this Jewish itinerant preacher was only written down much later and it is full of exaggerated myths and miracles. All information about him is based on oral traditions that were eventually (e.g., in the Gospels) written down. There are a few historical descriptions of him (e.g., by the Roman-Jewish historian Flavius Josephus or Tacitus), but they are sparse and not very meaningful.

Jesus probably never referred to himself directly as God, and yet he has remained as God in the cultural memory of humanity and became the founder of a world religion. How could this happen?

Here is a spotlight-like chronology of the most important events:

- Ca. 250 BC: The Greek version of the Hebrew Old Testament (OT) is written in Palestine ("Septuagint")
- 4 BC: probable year of birth of Jesus
- 29 AD: probable date of the crucifixion of Jesus
- 64: Persecution of Christians in Rome by Nero
- Around 65: Creation of the 1st Gospel (Mark)

- 325: Council of Nicaea establishes central foundations of Christian doctrine (only from this date is Jesus consistently regarded as God)
- 337: Constantine the Great converts to Christianity on his deathbed
- 386: Jerome writes the "Vulgate" (translation of the Bible into Latin)
- 401: Pope Innocent I claims worldwide supremacy for the Roman Church (later: Vatican)
- 484–519: first schism between West (Roman) and East (later Orthodox) Church
- 772: Charlemagne declares Christianity the religion of the Franks
- 1096–1099: 1st Crusade (of a total of 7)
- 1517: Beginning of the Reformation with Martin Luther's 95 Theses: Two confessional camps emerge: Catholics and Protestants
- 1618–1648: 30-year religious war between Catholicism and Protestantism
- July 17, 1870: 1st Vatican Council under Pius IX: From this point on, the Pope is considered infallible (when he speaks "ex cathedra")
- Etc.

References

Baumann, P., Uhlig, H.: Rettet die Naturvölker, Frankfurt 1980 (Fischer-TB)

Bothe, Hans-Werner, Engel, Michael: Die Evolution entlässt den Geist des Menschen, Frankfurt 1983 (Umschau)

Boetzkes, M. et al. (eds.): Eiszeit – Das große Abenteuer der Naturbeherrschung, Hildesheim 1999 (Roemer- und Pelizaeus-Museum)

Barrow, John D.: Der kosmische Schnitt – die Naturgesetze des Ästhetischen, Heidelberg/Berlin 1997 (Spektrum)

Bohm, David: Die implizite Ordnung – Grundlagen des dynamischen Holismus, München 1985 (Dianus/Trikont)

Eibl-Eibesfeldt, Irenäus: Der Mensch – das riskierte Wesen. Zur Naturgeschichte menschlicher Unvernunft, München 1988 (Piper)

Engels, Friedrich: Der Anteil der Arbeit an der Menschwerdung des Affen, Berlin 1986, 21th edn. (Dietz)

Haken, Hermann: Erfolgsgeheimnisse der Natur – Synergetik: Die Lehre vom Zusammenwirken, Stuttgart 1981 (DVA)

Jelinek, Jan; Das große Bilderlexikon des Menschen in der Vorzeit, Gütersloh 1972 (Bertelsmann)

Kanitscheider, Bernulf: Das Weltbild des Albert Einstein, München 1988 (Beck)

Karweina, Günther: Der sechste Sinn der Tiere, Hamburg 1982 (Stern/Gruner + Jahr)

Kuckenburg, Martin: Wer sprach das erste Wort? Die Entstehung von Sprache und Schrift, Darmstadt 2016 (Wissenschaftliche Buchgesellschaft)
Konner, Melvin: Die unvollkommene Gattung, Basel/Boston/Stuttgart 1983 (Birkhäuser)
Logan, Kevin: Crashkurs: Schöpfung und Evolution, Wuppertal 2004 (Brockhaus)
Leakey, Richard E.: Die Suche nach dem Menschen, Frankfurt 1981 (Umschau)
Morris, Richard: Darwins Erbe, Hamburg 2002 (Europa)
Roszak, Theodore: Das unvollendete Tier, München 1982 (trikont/dianus)
Schmitz, R., Thissen, J.: Neandertal – die Geschichte geht weiter, Heidelberg/Berlin 2000 (Spektrum)
Sheldrake, Rupert: Der siebte Sinn des Menschen, München 2003 (Scherz)
Samples, Bob: Der Geist der Mutter Erde – Ganzheitlichkeit und planetares Bewusstsein, Basel 1983 (Sphinx)
Todt, Dietmar: Das Leben – Werden und Vergehen, Gütersloh 1972 (Bertelsmann)
Vivelo, Frank Robert: Handbuch der Kulturanthropologie, Stuttgart 1981 (Klett-Cotta)
Wilber, Ken: Halbzeit der Evolution, Frankfurt 1996 (Fischer)
Wendt, Herbert: Der Affe steht auf, Reinbek 1971 (Rowohlt)
Weinreb, Friedrich: Wie sie den Anfang träumten, Bern 1976 (Origo)

Left

Die wichtigsten Göttinnen und Götter im Hinduismus (yogaeasy.de) (Stand: 18.09.2023)

6

A Power Greater than Ourselves: Conceptions of God

> **Summary**
>
> This chapter deals with the various conceptions of God and/or of gods and images of God. What attributes can be attributed to him/them? Is there a personal God—or are we dealing with impersonal energy(ies) and forces? How can one recognize him/them? Are there proofs of God—and what do they look like? Or is all this "religious humbug"? Is God only a "product of thought" and "wishful thinking" or is God—as Nietzsche writes—long dead and religion "opium for the people" (Marx)?
>
> It is not so long ago that a large part of people had time to think about themselves and the meaning of their lives and to consider who they are, what their soul is and what they are here for. It also deals with what the world is, what the cosmos is—and what God is. In earlier times, these questions were rather left to the priests or philosophers (in other cultures the shamans, gurus or mullahs) and their power of definition was trusted and their views were only too gladly adopted.

6.1 Is there God/Gods or only Images of God?

*"The success of dear God
is related to the fact,
that one does not <u>see</u> him."*

Dear God is also not what he once was. In the childhood of our personal life history, God was perhaps the "wise old man with the long beard". Later, the image of God gradually changed. Many of us have somehow completely lost him or we have lost sight of him—except in times of crisis. For some people, God is just a word, behind which something diffuse is located as a projection surface in the sound and smoke. So are God and heaven only something for child souls? And is there still something like his adversary (devil, Satan, Beelzebub) for us today? Just as the ideas of heaven have become more realistic, it is also true for many that the devil used to be more terrifying and hell was hotter. And the hereafter is also not what we once imagined.

God is a big word—and what individual people understand by it is highly different: For some, God is a force giving security, for others a judge and for others a complaint office …

6.2 The Multitude of Gods (Names)

The various religions are like the different languages. There is not a "good" and a "bad" language. But there is my language and your language. And I can get to know mine precisely and strive to learn other languages so that I can speak them without an accent. The messages that I express with the languages are something completely different. As described in the chapter about the past gods, there was and is an almost infinite number of conceptions of God with the most diverse names: God, Allah, YHWH ("Yahweh"), Manitou, TAO …

> *"The gods are our children,
> not our parents."*
> *(Balinese wisdom)*

In Hinduism alone, there are several hundred gods, with the three most famous being Brahma ("Creator"), Vishnu ("Preserver") and Shiva ("Destroyer") (for more on this, see: Chap. 5).

In monotheistic Islam, there is only one God, but there are still 99 names of Allah: Al-Rahiim = the Merciful, Al-Chaaliq = the Creator, Al-Rahman = the Compassionate, Al-Malik = the Lord, Al-Qudduus = the Holy, Al-Muhaymin = the Protector, Al-Aziiz = the Mighty, etc.

In Christianity, the concept of the triune God is held: Father, Son, and Holy Spirit ("Trinity"). God the Father is considered the creator of the universe and life. The Son is Jesus Christ, the God who became man. The Holy Spirit is understood as the spiritual life energy ("Ruach").

Before Christianity took over power in our cultural circle, there were also a multitude of gods here—Odin, Thor, Freya, Sol, and Tyr were their names, for example, among the Germanic peoples. And also in the Greek Olympus, besides the main gods—Zeus, Poseidon, Hera, Athena, and Hermes—there were several (also) regional gods, all of whom had human characteristics.

What can be said is: God is—if he exists at all—neither Catholic nor Protestant. He is not a Hindu or a Muslim, not a Jew or a Buddhist.

In our cultural circle, the three major monotheistic images of God prevail. In Christianity, Islam, and Judaism, one image of God is assumed. For monotheists, there is only one God—even if (at least in our cultural circle) fewer and fewer believe in it. In general, it can be said that the monotheistic religions are mostly "father religions" and have displaced or even destroyed the (female, mostly polytheistic) "mother religions" of the past.

6.3 Concepts of God

*"God is the place,
where all contradictions converge,
because they are resolved."
(Nicholas of Cusa)*

What do we actually mean when we talk about God? Does he exist or not? Is there only one God or several? And if so, are they a (or several) personal entity(ies) or impersonal energies or forces? Can we even comprehend these higher powers? Are the images and symbols of God that are still valid today, from several hundred or thousand years ago, still valid for our psyche today?

There are an infinite number of individual concepts of God:

- For some, God is the individual projection surface for the thoroughly good
- For others, God is absolute consciousness
- God is everything and nothing—and everything in between
- God is the indescribable One
- Since he is invisible, God has the advantage that he can be located anywhere: on the mountain, in the sky, on the earth, in the tree
- The sanctification of God is preached everywhere in religions, but it mainly happens in the mind of the respective person
- For some, he is the helmsman of life
- For others, he is the "good gardener" of life
- For many, he is an ordering force that provides orientation and structure
- For some, he is the lovingly patient God

- For others, he is the judging and punishing God
- For some, he is a bookkeeper God (all evil and good deeds are precisely registered)
- For others, he is a God of revenge and jealousy or even a war God
- For some, God is the "unmoved mover"
- And for others, God is a redemption machine or a complaint office
- For many, God serves as a kind of "filler", as a joint sealant and gap filler for everything that cannot be explained in this world. Where scientific evidence is lacking, God is used. In this sense, he is a kind of "multi-purpose God" or even "cosmic glue"
- Etc.

"God will forgive me,
it's his job."
(Heinrich Heine's last sentence
on his deathbed)

6.4 The Incarnation of God

Christians, for example, believe that with Jesus, God became human and wanted/should save us humans. But what does that actually mean – the incarnation of God? How should one imagine this? Does the good Lord think, "Oh, let's send these lost human souls some help so they know why they are here in the world—and who can explain it to them"? A somewhat childish idea—but (more or less consciously) it is not so rarely represented. Similar to the following idea:

"During the week, God lives in heaven.
Only on Sunday does he come to church."
(from a school essay)

And there are not only childish ideas about religion and God among children. Some remain lifelong and run through the entire history of religion: So do not confuse the good Lord with Santa Claus.

Even a Pope from the House of Medici, Leo X, made fun of the incarnation of God in the 16th century: "How much the fable of Christ has benefited us and ours is known."

The whole thing becomes problematic when this "revelation" of the truth is represented with a claim to absoluteness, which—because it was proclaimed in the respective holy book—allows no doubt about this dogma.

What many also forget: Christianity is an "imported religion" for our Central European culture from the Near East. Even in the Protestant Church, which likes to call itself a religion of reason, it says: Man did not create himself, but he is a creature of God. If one—as Luther did—assumes that every human being belongs to his creator and preserver, then he owes this living God thanks, praise, service, and obedience.

6.5 God—Attempts at Definition

"We can only say about God,
what he is not."
(Plotinus)

According to most philosophers of religion, God is indeed undefinable ("The God that exists does not exist," says Dietrich Bonhoeffer), but nevertheless the term God is regularly used and constantly talked about. And descriptions of him can be found everywhere:

He is considered the highest, almighty, all-knowing, eternal, uncreated, and supernatural being, which is not really tangible (nameless and indescribable). He is the infallible ruler of the universe, creator of heaven and earth, world creator and world ruler. Especially in monotheism, God is the personalized embodiment of the good, the force of nature, and the moral-spiritual power.

"God is the measure of all things."
(Bernard of Clairvaux)

For many religiously oriented philosophers, God is rather a principle—the basis on which reason ultimately stumbles. Since God is hidden or invisible, i.e., one cannot see him directly but only his works, he is—psychologically speaking—an infinite projection surface for everything that is good and positive. For God is—per definitionem—the infinitely good (more on this see further below: Proofs of God).

Does he now exist as a personal being—or are these only ideas that we make of him—i.e., images of God? And what is the use of a personalized God?

6.6 Advantages of a Personal God (Image)

It is certain—a personalized image of God facilitates many because they can enter into dialogue with it: Asking, Praying, Accusing, Demanding. With impersonal concepts of God (nature, energies, etc.), one cannot enter into dialogue. One is more or less at their mercy according to the motto "Either you stick to the rules or you will feel the results".

6.7 Characteristics of God

"God has no where"
"He is everything in all."
(Heinrich Sense, Mystic 1295–1366)

In monotheistic religions, God is attributed with a multitude of characteristics. Accordingly, he is omnipotent, omniscient, a structuring force, he brings order to life, is infinite, has no beginning and no end, is eternal. He is not seriously describable and not really comprehensible, because he is a supernatural being, embodiment of the good and highest authority.

In polytheistic religions, the individual gods are embodiments of certain characteristics. In Hinduism, for example, Saraswati is the goddess of wisdom, Krishna the embodiment of joy of life, and Lakshmi the goddess of prosperity.

Although the images of God are so blurred and diffuse, the monotheistic priests constantly talk about God in their sermons, and they act as if they already know what God is and what he wants.

6.8 What God has been used and misused for

God is just a word and he is by definition good—why is the world so bad?

In the beginning there was darkness and chaos. God created order and structure through the laws of nature, so the biblical idea, as believed by many.

As long as God remains vague and diffuse and only serves as a projection surface for the good, it usually still goes well. The problems always arise when the image of God is supposed to become concrete. What God has been misused for (small selection):

- How many people (e.g. witches) were tortured in the name of God?
- How many killings and murders (burning of heretics and witches) were committed in God's name?
- How many weapons and wars were blessed?
- How many (religious) wars were fought in his name?
- How many forced conversions were carried out?
- Etc.

Without God—if he exists—having resisted and sent a signal: Stop misusing my name all the time!!!

> **Heretical question** What reason is there to praise the Lord? For this world?

6.9 Theodicy: Why does God allow so much suffering and injustice?

"God died in Auschwitz."
(Theodor W. Adorno)

Behind theodicy is the following question: Why does an omniscient and omnipotent God allow so much evil in the world?

Gottfried Wilhelm Leibniz believes, if God were a "just judge", could he then allow so much unjustified suffering and evil in the world? In his text "On the Goodness of God, the Freedom of Man and the Origin of Evil" he considers how God's omnipotence and omniscience are compatible with the **free will of man,** i.e. also that man can "do evil". His result: God only wanted the good, but with human free will he also allowed evil. Therefore, all evil comes exclusively from man. God just allows it…

"I hope for His sake,
that God does not exist -
otherwise he would have to answer a lot of questions."
(Philip K. Dick)

6.10 Reason and Faith—Proofs of God

Can God be proven? Throughout the history of religion, there have always been numerous attempts to prove God. The most famous are presented here. Especially in today's science-believing times, this seems to be an important topic.

6.10.1 Anselm of Canterbury (1033–1109)

His goal was to restore the unity of faith and reason. Anselm seeks a rational justification for absolute faith and believes that no one should have to believe anything without some evidence: "I believe in order to understand." Already 700 years earlier, Augustine, the great Church Father, had formulated a similar sentence: "We believe in order to recognize." Even then, faith came first—and reason second.

For Anselm, God is something beyond which nothing greater can be thought. He is the all-powerful, perfect being who knows everything and can do everything. This is called the **ontological** proof of God.

In his view, there must be a God, because what does not exist is not perfect and we could not imagine God if he did not exist.

6.10.2 Thomas Aquinas (1225–1274)

The "Prince of Philosophers", the main representative of Scholasticism, is revered as a saint in the Catholic Church. He finds rational reasons for the existence of God. This is called the **cosmological** proof of God. His thesis: Nothing can be the cause and effect of itself. Therefore, the existence of the universe proves that the universe must have an external cause—and that is God. He therefore described "five ways to God", on which one finds God (which would also prove that he exists):

1. From the perspective of motion (God is for him the "unmoved mover")
2. From the perspective of the efficient cause (God is the first "efficient cause")
3. From the possible to the necessary (Every necessary thing has a cause coming from outside. And that is God)
4. From the perspective of degrees (There are things that are more or less good, true, and noble. But the perfectly good is God)
5. From the purposeful direction of things (They did not arise by chance, but there is a rational knowing that should reach its goal with purposeful intention. And that is God)

6.10.3 Nicholas of Cusa (1401–1464)

God is everything at once: He is the unity of opposites—cold and hot, soft and hard, merciful and cruel. But he is also contained in all earthly things.

The dual nature of God is inaccessible to human understanding: "God is greater than he can be understood." God eludes the grasp of human reason. Man has a common measure with God. Man can only find faith through "learned ignorance."

6.10.4 Thomas More (1478–1535)

He was the first philosopher to call his vision of the future "Utopia". On the island of Utopia (Greek: "place that does not exist") that he invented, people lived peacefully and carefree—almost like in paradise. The central orientations of the religiously tolerant Utopians were faith in God and the immortality of the soul. Utopia was something like the model for the legendary Atlantis or the mystical Avalon.

6.10.5 René Descartes (1596–1650)

For him, the path to knowledge was doubt. His most famous sentence "I think, therefore I am" summarizes the self-assurance through reflective thinking well. He is thus the founder of philosophical rationalism and epistemology. His proof of God looks like this: "When I think of God, I grasp that existence belongs to his essence, because he possesses all perfection." One could not think of God if he did not exist.

6.10.6 Blaise Pascal (1623–1662)

Pascal was a physicist, philosopher, and mathematician (pioneer of probability theory—some therefore say he was the inventor of roulette and the founder of "game theory"). For him, betting was the game of games. In his opinion, the "incomprehensibility of God" eludes human knowledge and understanding. Nevertheless, he recommends believing in God. The background can be represented in a kind of bet:

- What happens if I **do not** believe in God and he does not exist?
- What happens if I believe in God, even though he **does not** exist?
- What happens if I believe in God and he does exist?
- What happens if I **do not** believe in God, but he does exist?

"It is definitely worth believing in God and following his commandments. If God exists, it will pay off at the Last Judgment, if not, nothing is lost" (Blaise Pascal).

The lesser risk for Pascal is therefore to believe in God—thus one avoids the possible hell or purgatory. Tenor: "If you win, you win everything, and if you lose, you lose nothing … Without God, people only have distraction."

6.10.7 Baruch Spinoza (1632–1677)

Spinoza fled with his Jewish parents from the Inquisition in Portugal to Holland, where he (a few years later) was himself expelled from the Jewish community for "heresy" because he had and spread other, namely pantheistic, ideas of faith and God. He assumed an infinite, self-existing, eternal, and unchangeably absolute substance that stands behind everything visible and was God for him. He tried to approach and prove this substance through philosophy and reason. For him, this pantheistic view is an "ontological proof of God". Spinoza believed that philosophy should always be committed to the truth, and he radically separated it from theology, which he did not consider a science. This also made him a heretic.

6.10.8 Gottfried Wilhelm Leibniz (1646–1716)

If God were a "just judge" (Psalm 7), how could he allow so much unjustified suffering and evil in the world? This "theodicy" was primarily dealt with by Leibniz. In his text "On the Goodness of God, the Freedom of Man, and the Origin of Evil" (1705), he discusses the question of how God's omnipotence and omniscience can be reconciled with human free will, i.e., also that man can "do evil". His result: We live in the best of all worlds, where everything is possible. God only wanted the good, but with human free will, he also allowed evil. All evil therefore comes exclusively from humans, not from God.

6.10.9 Voltaire (Birth name: François-Marie Arouet, 1694–1778)

He was actually not an atheist, but a believer in God. However, he considered religious fanaticism to be much more problematic than godlessness. His favorite opponent was the Church, which he repeatedly covered with ironic-biting comments and ridiculed.

6.10.10 Immanuel Kant (1724–1804)

Kant (re-)discovered the categorical imperative: "Act in such a way that the maxim of your will could always simultaneously serve as the principle of general legislation." Although he often dealt with the question of God, Kant made it easy for himself in this regard: He said that the existence of God could not be proven from principled considerations with reasonable and logical arguments. Some therefore call him the "demolisher of proofs of God" or the "all-destroyer of metaphysics". In addition to dealing with the nature of God, the freedom of the will, and the immortality of the soul, he was primarily concerned with four important questions: "What can I know?", "What should I do?", "What may I hope for?" and "What is man?", with which he dealt in his works "Critique of Pure Reason", "Critique of Practical Reason", "Critique of Judgment", "Groundwork of the Metaphysics of Morals" etc. Although God cannot be proven, Kant recommends—for whatever reasons—to believe in him: "Two things fill the mind with ever new admiration and awe: The starry sky above me and the moral law within me."

6.10.11 Georg Wilhelm Friedrich Hegel (1770–1831)

Hegel originally wanted to explore God's fate before the creation of the world. Later, he described the state as an "appearing God", with which religion and politics were to be reconciled. In general, he was concerned with the reconciliation (or sublation) of opposites at a higher level:

"Thesis—Anti-Thesis > Synthesis."

For him, there was the progressing "world spirit", which continued to develop and was something like God on earth for him.

6.10.12 Arthur Schopenhauer (1788–1860)

For him, human life was a vale of tears: Whoever lives, suffers. The causes of suffering are desire and fear. Schopenhauer adopted many aspects of Buddhism, and—like most Buddhists—he had no concrete image of God. His life goal was to finally be able to step out of the wheel of rebirth ("Samsara") and sink into eternal nothingness.

6.10.13 Sören Kierkegaard (1813–1855)

The Danish philosopher was the first existentialist—long before Nietzsche, Sartre, and de Beauvoir. For him, man is a deficient being, subjected to the meaninglessness of existence and the arbitrariness of fate. He finds the way out of this isolation only through the three-stage process of turning to the aesthetic, the ethical self-determination of the individual, and then in the abolition of guilt and regret in religious overcoming and turning to God.

6.10.14 Friedrich Nietzsche (1844–1900)

For Nietzsche, man is a deficient being that must overcome itself. He should become something new, stronger by his own power: To become "superhuman", man must kill God. "Man is a rope tied between beast and superman—a rope over an abyss" (Thus Spoke Zarathustra). His most famous sentence is probably: "God is dead" (Nietzsche). In a graffiti at the Frankfurt University, someone had sprayed underneath: "Nietzsche is dead" (God).

6.10.15 Bertrand Russell (1872–1970)

The philosopher and founder of the "antinomy" named after him says: "I am convinced that there is no nonsense that a government could not persuade its subjects to believe." And this attitude, the atheist and rationalist Russell also has towards religion: "If everything must have a cause, then God must also have a cause."

6.10.16 Karl Jaspers (Psychiatrist, Philosopher, 1883–1969)

Throughout his life, man is exposed to existential crises and boundary situations that are difficult to comprehend—suffering, fear, guilt, struggle, fate, death, which everyone must cope with in their own way. This happens out of fear of failure by a leap to self-being and thus to the feeling of freedom and self-responsibility. Jaspers refers to this leap as "transcendence", as "philosophical faith" or sometimes also as "God".

6.10.17 Albert Camus (1913–1960)

According to an ancient Greek legend, Sisyphus had outwitted death several times. Because he was a sinner, he was condemned by the gods to a senseless punishment: He must push a heavy boulder up a mountain for all eternity. And—just before he reaches the top, the rock slips from his hand and tumbles down and he has to start all over again. For Camus, this was in his work "The Myth of Sisyphus" (1942) the symbol for the absurdity and meaninglessness of human life: "One must imagine Sisyphus happy."

In his novel "The Plague" he calls the plague a just punishment and the "flail of God". He does not pose the theodicy, the question of the just God, but Camus is an explicit atheist.

6.10.18 Jean-Paul Sartre (1905–1980)

Sartre writes in his diary: "One must be made of clay, and I am made of wind." He simply was not tough enough for the hardships of life and thus finds himself in the tradition of the early existentialists (Spinoza, Kierkegaard, Husserl). In his main work "Being and Nothingness" (1943), Sartre emerges as the most radical philosopher of freedom. Like Camus, he believes: We humans are **condemned to freedom** and must be our own saviors. No God (which for these existentialists does not exist anyway) and no religion can help. Man is born—according to Sartre's view—as raw mass and must give himself a form—if he does not do this, he is shaped from the outside. That's why he also resists the religious view, because in the Christian religion the responsibility is shifted to the transcendent: "God wills it so." With the result that tens of thousands were murdered in the name of God. As the Crusaders did to the Cathars in Languedoc on the orders of the Pope in the 13th century. Motto: "Kill them all—God will recognize his own."

"Even gods die,
when no one believes in them."
(Jean-Paul Sartre)

6.10.19 Ludwig Wittgenstein (1881–1951)

The world is the totality of all facts. We form our thoughts about the facts of the world in words and sentences. When one speaks about things not directly visible (e.g., God or soul), these are for Wittgenstein "empty sentences": "Whereof one cannot speak, thereof one must be silent," is one of his most famous sentences. However, the language analyst Wittgenstein writes in his philosophical diaries of a "conformity with the world" or of that "alien will," on which we depend and which we call God. And Wittgenstein's ambivalence towards the topic of religion is evident in another conversation: "I am not a religious person, but I cannot help it: I see every problem from a religious standpoint."

6.10.20 Hans Küng (1928–2021)

The Swiss theologian was a professor at the Eberhard Karls University in Tübingen from 1960 to 1996. He founded the "Project World Ethos" in 1990 and has written many books. One of the most important is called "Does God Exist?". In it, he distinguishes between external and internal rationality:

- He understands **"external rationality"** to mean that "the hidden reality of God does not impose itself on reason," so the rational recognition of God is not in the foreground.
- The **"internal rationality"** provides something like a fundamental certainty: "In the act of daring trust in God's reality, man experiences, despite all temptation by doubt, the reasonableness of his trust: founded in a final identity, meaningfulness and value of reality, in its primal ground. Original sense, primal value" (p. 630).

6.10.21 Dorothee Sölle (1929–2003)

"Believe in God atheistically?", Dorothee Sölle, a contentious evangelical feminist theologian, asked. Is that possible? To believe atheistically? Can one believe in something that does not exist? God has been declared dead time and again—not only by Nietzsche—but rarely by theologians. When Dorothee Sölle, a conflict-capable and energetically devout theologian, declared God dead at the Protestant Church Congress in 1965, it was quite a small revolution. Sölle was a politically engaged and church-provoking mystic. In her book "Believe in God Atheistically" (Walter-Verlag, Olten 1968), she demanded a radical departure from the omnipotent patriarchal image of a God who has everything under control and regulates everything:

"Where was God in Auschwitz?", she writes: "Why didn't he stop the trains? If he can do everything?" Later she writes in her memoirs: "I just wanted to say that we need God, but not the Fitzliputzli who arranges everything from above." For her, God is far away. He does not care. He does not exist in the form many imagine him. She says: "God needs us." He needs the help of people to become visible and recognizable. In her later work, she no longer assumes a personal God, but wants to "believe in God atheistically".

That she cannot make a professional career with such an attitude within the established church theologian hierarchy is understandable. Although she can complete her habilitation at the University of Cologne, a professorship at a German university remains denied to her. She does teach at the Union Theological Seminary in New York from 1975 to 1987 and has individual teaching assignments at German universities, but she cannot make a career within the German church—like so many who stray from the mainstream of the flock.

The Jesuit priest and Zen master Niklaus Brantschen has only recently published a book that represents a similar attitude. It is called "Praying without God" (Ostfildern 2022, Patmos-Verlag).

6.10.22 Robert Spaemann (1927–2018)

He was a professor of philosophy at the University of Heidelberg from 1969 to 1992. In 2007, he published the book "The Last Proof of God," which is based on an earlier lecture titled "The Reasonableness of Belief in God." However, he does not believe in reason, not in scientism, the purely scientific explanation of our existence. His thesis is: "Truth presupposes God" and for "eternal truths absolute consciousness—i.e., God—is necessary". "Believing that God is, means that he is not our idea, but that we are his idea. It therefore means a reversal of perspective—conversion."

6.10.23 Kurt Gödel (1906–1978)

The Austrian mathematician presented a mathematical proof of God, according to which God necessarily exists, whose contradiction-free chain of argument was even confirmed by scientists from the Free University of Berlin and the TU Vienna in 2013.

6.10.24 Viktor Frankl (1905–1997): The Unconscious God

The Austrian psychiatrist Viktor Frankl writes in his book "The Unconscious God": "The unconscious belief of man that is thus revealed … would mean that God has always been unconsciously intended by us, that we have always had an intentional relationship with God, even if unconscious. And we call this God the unconscious God. Our formula of the unconscious God does not mean that God himself, for himself, is unconscious; rather, it means that God is sometimes unconscious to us, that our relation to him can be unconscious, namely repressed and thus hidden from ourselves."

Already in the Psalms, there is talk of the "hidden God" and in Hellenistic antiquity there was an altar dedicated to the "unknown God" (Frankl. The Unconscious God, pp. 55–56).

"The success of the dear God is related to the fact that one does not see him."

"God is the only being that,
to rule,
does not even have to exist."
(Charles Baudelaire)

6.10.25 Proofs of God: Conclusio

And this is just a small selection of attempts to prove—or disprove—God. But what are proofs of God? The fact that the proofs of God are sometimes logical circular arguments is just briefly mentioned here. They are certainly not what one would accept as proof in the natural sciences or mathematics—they are not controllable and independent of the subject/objective. Because they are open to various interpretations—and one must believe them—since God is invisible—(or just leave it). So they are more like theses than proofs in the scientific sense. At least: God remains silent about it.

"Reason can only touch God,
but never grasp him."
(Albertus Magnus, 1200–1280)

6.11 Belief and Knowledge: The Critical Voices

"If only I could feel,
that God loves me.
But he never tells me."
(Charles de Foucauld)

But there were already very early attempts (e.g., among the ancient Greeks) to describe God and gods—what they are and what they are not. Already then, it was about the confrontation between belief and knowledge: What do I know for sure and what do I have to believe? Because even then there were critical voices, sometimes with the aim of deconstructing the gods. Especially with a view to the panopticon of the ancient Greek gods in Olympus, the philosopher Xenophanes (ca. 580–480 BC) criticized more than 2500 years ago that many religions imagined their gods like humans: "If horses had gods, they would probably look like horses." Which was of course a blasphemous attack on the then (as now) understanding of gods. But also Protagoras (485–415 BC) turned the conceptions of gods upside down: Not the gods had made the people, but the people had made the gods. And thus, they were something like the ancestors of later critics of religion, such as:

- Ludwig Feuerbach (1804–1872): "God is a product of thought and a wishful thinking of man."
- Karl Marx (1818–1883): "Religion is opium for the people."
- Friedrich Nietzsche (1844–1900): "God is dead."
- Sigmund Freud (1856–1939): "Religion is an obsessive-compulsive disorder."

"If there were no God, one would have to invent him," Voltaire thought. *"Which has indeed been done,"* said the philosopher Diderot in conversation with him.

6.12 "World Soul" and "Sacred Matrix"

Is there perhaps no personal God, but something like a "World Soul"—as also represented by Hegel? It is rejected (or at least reinterpreted) by the Judeo-Christian belief in creation, but it has repeatedly appeared in pantheism. Especially in Romanticism, the World Soul was used as a metaphor for the interconnected vitality of nature. A similar term appears over two thousand years ago in Plato's writing "Timaeus", which deals with the nature of the world, the cosmos, and the search for the "world formula" as a whole. According to this, the cosmos was created as a rational, animated being by a benevolent creator, in which man exists as an animated cosmos in miniature and can only be happy if he lives in harmony with the laws of the cosmos and in unison with the World Soul.

The psychologist Dieter Duhm, one of the founders of the alternative project "Tamera" in Portugal, calls a very similar concept to the World Soul the "Sacred Matrix. In his book of the same name (Belzig, 2001, Meiga Publishing), he describes his ideas for the spiritual improvement of the world through communities of peace activists like Tamera and the establishment of so-called "healing biotopes".

6.13 The Scientific Perspective

"I thank the good Lord,
that he made me an atheist."
(Georg Christoph Lichtenberg)

In Islam it is said: "Allah is great and Mohammed is his prophet." An ironically oriented scientist made of it: "The universe is great and Haley is its comet." For many scientists, religion is not provable and the "soul" (or psyche) may be nothing more than the result of the experiences that a person has made on the basis of his genetic equipment and which are reflected as the result of electrical impulses in neurological pathways of the brain (for more on this see Chap. 11: Religious enlightenment experiences and altered states of consciousness). For a theologian or spiritually oriented philosopher, the soul may be an immortal entity that is possibly reborn in a new body again and again (reincarnation).

6.14 Conclusion

One cannot prove that God exists—but also not that he *does not* exist. God is therefore a kind of hypothesis. It is verified by some, falsified by others—depending on the starting position. The reality of God arises in the eye of the beholder. If the observer is a believer, he can see him everywhere. For unbelievers, he is not present.

Is it therefore perhaps better to remain silent about God, rather than to talk about him?

"The **small** truth has many words.
The **great** truth has only silence."
(Buddhist wisdom)

References

Brantschen, Niklaus: Gottlos beten, Ostfildern 2022 (Patmos-Verlag)
Bochenski, I. M.: Die zeitgenössischen Denkmethoden, München 1954 (UTB-Francke)
Blume, R. G., Kropfberger, K.: Homo systemicus, Göttingen 2020 (Vandenhoeck und Ruprecht)
Bucher, Anton A.: Psychologie der Spiritualität, Weinheim 2007 (Beltz)
Duhm, Dieter: Heilige Matrix, Belzig, 2001 (Verlag Meiga)
Federspiel, K., Lackinger-Karger, I.: Kursbuch Seele, Köln 1996 (Kiepenheuer + Witsch)
Frankl, Viktor E.: Der Wille zum Sinn – Bern 1972, 2. Auflage (Huber)
Frankl, Viktor E.: Die Sinnfrage in der Psychotherapie, München 1981 (Piper)
Hellinger, Bert: Religion, Psychotherapie, Seelsorge, München 2000 (Kösel)
Schlette, Heinz Robert: Weltseele – Geschichte und Hermeneutik, Frankfurt 1993 (Knecht)
Huisman, Denis: Philosophie für Einsteiger, Reinbek 1983 (Rowohlt)
Janich, Peter: Was ist Erkenntnis?, München 2000 (C.H. Beck)
Küstenmacher, M. et al.: Gott 9.0 – wohin unsere Gesellschaft spirituell wachsen wird, Gütersloh 2010, (Gütersloher Verlagshaus)
Küng, Hans: Existiert Gott?, Freiburg 2017 (Herder)
Metz, Wulf (Eds.): Handbuch Weltreligionen, Wuppertal 2003 (Brockhaus)
Nozick, Robert: Vom richtigen, guten und glücklichen Leben, München 1993 (DTV)
Sölle, Dorothee: Atheistisch an Gott glauben, Olten/CH 1968 (Walter)
Utsch, M., Bonelli, R. M., Pfeifer, S.: Psychotherapie und Spiritualität, Berlin/Heidelberg 2014 (Springer)
Wahl, Francois (Eds.): Einführung in den Strukturalismus, Frankfurt 1973 (Suhrkamp)
Wittgenstein, Ludwig: Philosophische Untersuchungen, Frankfurt 1971 (Suhrkamp)

7

How the Holy Books became Holy: Their Origin and Function

> **Summary**
> The following chapter describes the origin of the so-called Holy Books—Bible, Torah, Quran, etc.—and how they became sacred. It explains how the process goes from oral traditions passed down over several generations to the transcription, canonization, and dogmatization—and thus also to the first intra-religious faith conflicts.
> In addition, the function of the Holy Books is presented. How do they provide orientation and support and help to align life accordingly? But also: Where do they become problematic dogma and—in the worst case—an argument to torture and kill people?

History is always also a collection of stories. And religions in particular are conglomerates of stories. First orally passed on from generation to generation (with all the subjective interpretations and adapted to the respective zeitgeist, cultural and societal conditions). Later then written down and at some point codified and canonized with a clear separation of what has to be true and right and what is wrong—and what is thus outside the belief system. In the Christian area, these are mainly the "Apocrypha"—the forbidden writings of the Bible (see below). So what is the right belief—and what is superstition? The holy books serve to draw a line of separation here.

Finally, there are a multitude of writings that were later declared sacred.

Several religions even claim that the Holy Books (Bible, Torah, Quran) were written by the respective God himself or directly given (or even dictated) to the prophet—or at least inspired by him.

7.1 From the Visions of the Prophets to Canonization

In reality, it probably looked more like the respective prophet had visions, fantasies or dreams that he took for God's inputs and that he communicated as truth to his disciples, students, adepts or the community as a whole. These were then passed on orally—and that from generation to generation—with all the extensions, dramatizations, exaggerations already mentioned above that are common in narratives. But this is also how myths and miracle stories are created—they become more and more wonderful the more often they are retold. At some point, they were written down. They were then fixed. And from then on the fight really started: What is the truth? What is right, what is exaggerated and wrong? What belongs in the Holy Books—and what does not? This is called "canonization"—so what belongs in the canon and what is sorted out. This could be seen particularly well in the Christian area with the "Apocrypha" (hidden books). These are the religious writings of Christian or Jewish origin that did not make it into the biblical canon.

The biblical canon is therefore the books that Judaism and Christianity have established as components of the "Holy Scripture" and thus made the standard of religious practice.

7.2 How and when was the Bible created?

The term "Bible" comes from Greek. The Greek "biblia" means "books" and is also found in the (german) word (Bibliothek) library. Because the Bible is actually **not just one** book, but a kind of library. Some therefore also refer to the Bible as the "book of books".

The Bible is divided into the "Old Testament" (OT) and the "New Testament" (NT) and these are again divided into various books or writings. The OT comprises 39 books and the NT is divided into 27 books. All texts were written at different times by different and unknown authors. However, these stories were previously passed on orally over many generations—with all the uncertainties and subjective accentuations that go along with oral traditions. From about the 9th century BC and until the 2nd century BC, the texts of the OT were fixed in writing. The Old Testament was written in Hebrew and consists of law books, history books, textbooks, psalms, and books of the prophets. Who wrote the original versions of the Bible is still unknown today. There are many gaps, puzzles, and contradictions in the traditions. According to many dogmatists, however, it is still God's word that has been passed on unadulterated.

Only this much is certain: The Holy Scriptures of the Jews, the **Tanakh,** is definitely what the Christians have adopted as the Old Testament (for more on this, see: 7.3 Torah, Talmud and Tanakh).

The New Testament was written in Greek and includes the four Gospels (= good news) of the Apostles Matthew, Mark, Luke, and John. The NT was written in the 1st century AD—long after the death of the evangelists. In addition, the NT in the Acts of the Apostles tells about the life of Jesus Christ, his work, his death, and the resurrection. In addition to this, the NT includes various letters from the apostles to their communities and the Revelation of John, which also deals with the apocalypse.

Until around 140 AD, the most important writings of the later New Testament are available, but there is no generally accepted selection. For even at this early time, various groups are competing for what the right Christianity should look like. However, it takes more than 200 years for the canon of the NT to be finally written down. Only in the year 367 AD is the New Testament limited to 27 writings. All other writings do not belong to what must be believed. The excluded writings—as already mentioned above—are called "Apocrypha".

The Bible is considered the foundation of two world religions—Judaism and Christianity. Over the past centuries, more than 5 billion Bibles have been printed worldwide in several hundred languages. Every year, another 30 million copies are added. However, it is not known how many of these are actually read. After all, about a third of the world's population is Christian (currently about 2.28 billion).

The Bible used to be considered the authentic "Word of God", and many church organizations assumed that God spoke directly through the Bible. Today—except in Christian sects—people have mostly moved away from calling it that. Today it is rather said that the Bible depicts experiences of God and what tasks God assigns to people. However, despite many oddities and inconsistencies, it is considered "Holy Scripture". After all, the Bible is full of oddities, errors, speculations, critical points, and untruths:

- Jesus was probably not born in Bethlehem, but likely in Nazareth.
- Jesus was not born at "Christ's birth", but between 4 and 6 BC.
- There is no evidence for Herod's murder of the innocent children.
- The census did not take place until around 75 AD.

- Joseph (the husband of Jesus' mother Mary) most likely did not come from the house of David (detailed genealogy from Adam to David), but from a family of craftsmen.
- John the Baptist, who announces Jesus as his successor, and Mary (Jesus' mother) did not know each other.
- Reinterpretations of the prophet Isaiah, who had announced Jesus already 700 years BC.
- Immaculate Conception: translation error (virgin and young woman).
- Jesus probably had siblings (James, Josos, Judas, Simon).
- Bodily Ascension of Jesus and Mary.
- Jesus probably looked very different from the image conveyed by the churches.
- No star that led the Three Wise Men from the East to Jesus' crib.
- Jesus has only been consistently referred to as God since the Council of Nicaea.

However, there is not "the Bible", but each church or religious organization has its own Bible. These different Bibles are the same in basic structure, but there are differences between the Catholic and the Protestant, between the Orthodox and, for example, the version of the Jehovah's Witnesses. Sometimes the differences are minimal (e.g., due to different translations and emphases), but sometimes the differences are also significant due to various interpretations.

The Catholic Bible consists of 73 books (46 OT and 27 NT). The Protestant Bible contains a total of 66 books (39 OT and 27 NT). "Sola scriptura", only the scripture (is the central anchor of faith). This core sentence of the Reformation, as Martin Luther is said to have said, does not have it easy with such uncertain scriptural conditions, however …

> **Heretical question** What is really holy about the "Holy Scripture" Bible?

7.3 Torah, Talmud, and Tanakh: The Foundations of Jewish Faith

Of the five major world religions, Judaism is considered the oldest continuous faith. It has existed for over 3,000 years. Jews are among the oldest peoples in human history. Jewish history is a history full of expulsions, struggles, victories, and defeats: Jews had to flee from Egypt, sought the "promised land", were expelled again, lived under Babylonian rule, their temple was destroyed and rebuilt …

At the beginning of Jewish history stands **Abraham,** who is something like the patriarch of the Jewish people. He is also considered the founder of monotheism, that is, the belief in a single God.

There are a multitude of central figures in Jewish history. The most important are (besides Abraham) **Moses** (who led the Jews out of Egyptian captivity and around 1230 BC is said to have received the 10 Commandments and the Torah from God on Mount Sinai), **David** (the later king of Israel, who defeated Goliath).

The most significant works of Judaism are:

- Torah (Teaching, Instruction)
- Tanakh (Bible)
- Talmud (Instruction)

The **Torah** in the narrower sense includes the five books of Moses. It is the main source of both Jewish law and Jewish ethics—and it formulates Jewish customs. So it not only establishes the religious aspects of life, but it is also identity-forming for being "Jewish"—that is, the way one should live as a Jew.

In a broader sense, however, the Torah also includes the entire Jewish Bible. This is the so-called Tanakh.

Believing Jews call their Bible namely **Tanakh.** The three consonants T—N—Kh stand for the three parts of the Jewish Bible: "Torah" (oral tradition), "Nevi'im" (Prophets) and "Ketuvim" (Writings).

The **Talmud** is—next to the Torah—the most important work of Judaism. It originated from oral traditions that were only later written down. The Talmud contains stories, sayings, and aids for coping with everyday life and various arguments. It consists of the **"Mishnah",** in which the laws from the Torah are collected, assigned, and interpreted in six areas. The **"Gemara"** provides extensive commentaries. The Talmud was formulated in its final version around 500 AD.

> **Heresy Objection**
>
> God said, "I have commandments for you."
> Moses asked, "And what do they cost?"
> "Nothing," God replied.
> "Then I'll take ten," Moses replied. (Jewish joke)

It is not quite easy to live according to the strict Jewish regulations (Mitzvot). For they are numerous and affect all possible aspects of life. In addition to the 10 Commandments, there are 613 Mitzvot in the Torah—including 365 prohibitions and 248 commandments.

The most well-known (among non-Jews) are the regulations for dealing with food. What can be eaten according to the Torah rules is called "kosher", what should not be eaten is called "trefe". So there are animals, that are kosher (e.g., ruminants like sheep or cows), while pigs are not ruminants and therefore not kosher. And the animals must be "slaughtered" when slaughtered, i.e., there must be no (liquid) blood left in the dead animal, as Jews are not allowed to eat blood. Reptiles, shellfish, or crustaceans are also not allowed to be eaten. Fish may only be eaten if they have fins and scales …

A special feature of Jewish dietary rules is, for example, the Kashrut regulation that milk and meat must not be stored, prepared, or eaten together. These guidelines may have had their (also health-protecting) sense hundreds of years ago, when there were many more widespread animal diseases, there were no preservation and cooling possibilities. Nowadays, the regulations are (medically speaking) mostly unnecessary and sometimes nonsensical. Apart from the religious, they usually have no more sense.

Here it becomes apparent how religious dogmatism can be rigidly outdated and lead to more or less nonsensical restrictions.

"Dogmas are like street lamps."
"They illuminate the path of the faithful."
"But only drunks cling to them."
(Karl Rahner, Theologian)

There are currently approximately 15.3 million Jews worldwide. Of these, 7.1 million live in Israel and about 6 million in the USA. Larger Jewish communities also exist in France, Canada, the United Kingdom, and Germany.

7.4 Origin and Significance of the Quran

Islam was founded approximately 1400 years ago. It is—like Judaism and Christianity—a monotheistic religion. Judaism, Christianity, and Islam are also called the "Abrahamic book religions" because they all regard Abraham as an early prophet and strictly adhere to their holy books (Bible, Torah, Quran).

Although Islam is a strictly monotheistic religion, there are 99 names of Allah: Al-Rahiim = the Merciful, Al-Chaaliq = the Creator, Al-Rahman = the Compassionate, Al-Malik = the Lord, Al-Qudduus = the Holy, Al-Muhaymin = the Protector, Al-Aziiz = the Mighty, etc.

After Christianity, Islam, with approximately 1.9 billion Muslims, is the second largest and fastest growing world religion. There are two important main branches in Islam—the Sunnis (approx. 85%) and the Shiites (approx. 15%), who do not always interact amicably with each other.

The holy book of Muslims is called the Quran (Qur'an). This book collects the texts that the Archangel Gabriel is said to have dictated to the Prophet Mohammed.

The Quran is divided into 114 chapters (suras) and approximately 6,666 verses. They tell of God and provide Muslims with rules on how to lead their lives. The revelations were received by Mohammed between 610 and 632 (AD). He received the first revelation in a cave on Mount Hira.

While in Christianity Jesus is seen as God (in Islam he is called Isa), in Islam he is just a prophet among other prophets (Noah, Abraham, Moses, and Mohammed).

Islamic faith rests on five pillars:

1. Profession of faith (Shahada)
2. Praying five times a day (Salat)
3. Fasting month (Ramadan)
4. Alms tax (Zakat)
5. Pilgrimage to Mecca (Hajj)

Islam claims—similar to Judaism—to provide clear guidelines to believers on how they should live. In addition to the Quran, in Islam, **Sunna** (established behaviors, traditions) and **Sharia** (severe penalties for "offenses against the divine order") regulate life.

What is called "kosher" in Judaism is called "halal" in Islam—that is, all that one should eat. The prohibitions (haram) particularly include the prohibition of alcohol and the prohibition of eating pork. But there are also regulations for many other areas of life, e.g., dress codes (e.g., headscarf, hijab, burka for women, prayer clothing/Jalabyia for men) or purification rules before prayer.

Since the Quran is regarded by Mohammed as a direct revelation from Allah (God), it must not be changed. However, as with Christianity, it was first passed on orally before it was written down long after Mohammed's death—with all the uncertainties described above.

7.5 Other Holy Books

Of course, in addition to the three book religions, there are a multitude of scriptures from other religions that are considered holy books. Virtually every religion has its own holy scripture. A holy book is considered in a religious community to set norms for members in matters of faith, ethical principles, and ritual questions. These guidelines are often used and quoted in cultic actions, services, and rituals. Often, the holy scriptures are also an expression of the teachings of the religion's founder and form a proper canon in well-structured religious communities. The respective holy scripture is treated with respect and reverence within the community. There are usually also the valid interpretations and interpretations of the scripture.

As it would go beyond the scope of this book, I will only briefly touch on a few other so-called holy books:

- In Hinduism, the "Bhagavad Gita", the "Vedas" and the "Puranas" are considered holy scriptures.
- In Buddhism, there are—depending on the orientation—several holy scriptures: In Theravada Buddhism it is the "Pali Canon", in Mahayana Buddhism it is the "Heart Sutra" and the "Lotus Sutra".
- In Taoism it is the "Tao Te Ching".
- For the Parsis (Zoroastrianism/Zarathustra), the holy book is called "Avesta".
- Etc.

> **Heresy Objection**
>
> In reality, there are no holy books. Holiness only arises in the mind and heart of the person.

(For more on this, see: 12. What is sacred to me …).

References[1]

Alexander, Pat und David: Das große Handbuch zur Bibel, Witten 2001 (SCM-Brockhaus)

---

[1] **Without literature references:** Bible (Judaism and Christianity), Quran (Islam), „Bhagavad Gita" (Hinduism), „Pali Canon" (Theravada Buddhism), „Heart Sutra" (Mahayana Buddhism), „Tao Te Ching" (Taoism), „Avesta" (Zoroastrianism), „Kitab-i-Aqdas" (Bahai).

Bork, Uwe: Kleines Lexikon biblischer Irrtümer, Gütersloh 2009 (Gütersloher Verlagshaus)
Koch, K. et al. (Eds.): Reclams Bibellexikon, Stuttgart 1992 (Reclam)
Mears, Henrietta: Alles was man über die Bibel wissen muss, Wuppertal 2004 (Brockhaus)
Metz, Wulf (Eds.): Handbuch Weltreligionen, Wuppertal 2003 (Brockhaus)
Ruffing, Reiner: Kleines Lexikon wissenschaftlicher Irrtümer, Gütersloh 2011 (Gütersloher Verlagshaus)
Satinover, Jeffrey: Die verborgene Botschaft der Bibel, München 1997 (Goldmann)
Schnepper, Arndt: Zankäpfel der Kirche Wuppertal 2007, (R.Brockhaus)
Vogel, Walter: Die Religionsstifter, Wiesbaden 2008 (Marix)

8

Gods, Prophets, Angels, Saints, and Priests: Who They are, What They Do, and What They Want

> **Summary**
>
> This chapter deals with the various actors in the religious field—from the gods over angels, saints and prophets to the "ground staff of God", i.e. the priests in the religions—regardless of whether they are called pastors, bishops, apostles, brahmins, mullahs, shamans, lamas, gurus or simply "clerics". Where are they the link, "channel" or bridge of the believers to faith and God? How do they help the religious community interpret the religious scriptures? When are they "representatives of God" on earth? How powerful are they? What advantages do they have in society?

"Man is a rope tied between beast and overman," Friedrich Nietzsche wrote almost 150 years ago. And the longing for the "overman" can manifest in many ways. Especially in the esoteric scene, the psycho market, and in some modern religions, the transitions between humans, prophets, angels, and gods seem to be fluid. There are people who claim to have a direct line to God ("channeling"), others say "God is in everything" and promise "you too can become divine". And yet others consider themselves to be representatives of God on earth—or angels.

8.1 Angels—Messengers between God and Man?

Angels were long an endangered species—currently, they are back in fashion.

The word "angel" comes from Hebrew and means "messenger". Angels are considered heavenly beings of mythological origin. They are messengers between man and God. In monotheistic religions (Judaism, Christianity, Islam), angels are seen as spiritual beings in human form. According to this view, they were created by God and are subordinate to him. Angels are said to be able to reveal God's messages and instructions to chosen people. Thomas Aquinas refers to angels as immaterial beings that consist of pure form and have no material dimension. For those who believe in angels, there is a whole heaven full of angels and a proper angel hierarchy:

Archangels hold a leading position within the host of angels. According to the Bible, there are seven archangels (Michael, Gabriel, Uriel, Raphael, Barachiel, Sealtiel, Jehudiel), who deliver far-reaching and important messages from God that affect entire nations—while the simple angels take care of individual people like you and me.

In addition, there are **"Cherubim"** and **"Seraphim"**, who guard the heavenly throne and the Garden of Eden. But there are also other heavenly angelic beings: judgment angels, malevolent angels, and even a death angel, who is called Azrael in Islam.

An important category of angels, well known to most religious people, are the **Guardian Angels.** They are considered lower angelic beings, but they experience a boom in our latitudes time and again. In recent years, there has been a recurring wave of a real guardian angel hype, in which the "heavenly poultry" not only brings a lot of money into the coffers of providers at esoteric fairs with angel figures, angel amulets, angel cards, and even angel perfume, but also the number of sayings about and with angels in religions is almost infinite:

- "An angel is someone God sends you to light up a few stars in the sky for you when things get tough and dark."
- "Of all the companions who accompanied me, none has remained as faithful to me as the guardian angel." (Clemens von Brentano)
- "I wish for an angel, I want to feel God's presence. Good angel come to me, to touch me tenderly."
- "The angels are very close to us and protect us and God's creatures on his behalf." (Martin Luther)
- "Never drive faster than your guardian angel can fly."
- "Fall and I will catch you. Cry and I will comfort you. Fight and I will fight with you."
- "Never stand at the foot of a sickbed. This place is always reserved for the guardian angel."

- "Do not go where your guardian angel cannot follow you."
- "May the angels accompany you to paradise."
- Etc.

But not only in Christianity, Judaism, and Islam are there angels, but similar intermediary beings also exist in other major religions. In Buddhism, these enlightened beings are called **Bodhisattvas,** in Hinduism they are called **Devas.**

Since these intermediary beings are spiritual beings not visible to all people, today's angel people are often portrayed as "avatars" on the internet and in cyberspace.

It is not certain whether these are primarily emotionally highly charged intrapsychic perceptions and processes that are triggered by the traditional and widespread angel mythology, or—in the worse case—religious fantasies. The discussion about angels is not new: Already in the Middle Ages, for example, there were long-lasting and seriously conducted philosophical discussions about how many angels could fit on the head of a pin …

8.2 Prophets: Proclaimers of Divine Truths

The word Prophet means "messenger", "advocate", "announcer". He is supposed to be a person through whom God speaks to people. Prophets exist in many religions. They mostly report encounters with God and proclaim His messages. Example: The 10 Commandments are said to have been given to the Prophet Moses by God on Mount Sinai.

Prophets admonish people to obey God's commandments, to refrain from idolatry (the gods of other religions were often declared idols and their priests defamed as idolaters). Prophets primarily appeal to the faithful to follow religious rules of life.

In the Christian-Jewish area, Abraham is considered the 1st prophet. In Judaism, the four major prophets are Isaiah, Jeremiah, Ezekiel, and Daniel, and the twelve minor prophets are Hosea, Joel, Amos, Obadiah, Jonah, Micah, Nahum, Habakkuk, Zephaniah, Haggai, Zechariah, Malachi.

In Islam, although Abraham is also considered a prophet, for Muslims, Adam is the 1st prophet. The Quran mentions 25 prophets (e.g., Adam, Noah, Abraham, Moses, Jesus). According to various sources, however, there should have been many more prophets in Islam. The Prophet Mohammed saw himself as a messenger of God. He is considered the last and greatest prophet and is therefore known as the "Seal of the Prophets". His revelations—as they are written down in the Quran—are considered by Muslims to be the unadulterated word of God and are a guide for an Islamic way of life. The person Mohammed is also considered a model for a just and virtuous life.

So far the historical prophets. What about today? In the end, there is no clear definition of prophets, because in recent years people like Mahatma Gandhi, Martin Luther King, Nelson Mandela, Oscar Romero, and Mother Teresa have been considered modern prophets.

And nowadays the esoteric market is full of people who—more or less admitted—consider themselves prophets: "When the sun of culture is quite low, dwarfs can appear like giants."

8.3 How People Became (Made into) Gods

In many earlier cultures, people could become gods and there were always transitions between god and man. The deification ("Apotheosis"), was present, for example, among the ancient Egyptians: Pharaohs were considered gods. The Sumerians regarded Gilgamesh as a god-king. Even Alexander the Great and Julius Caesar were attributed god-kingly qualities. To this day, the Emperor of Japan (Tenno) is considered a god.

But not only at the royal level does apotheosis occur: To this day, in Kathmandu (Nepal), "Kumaris" are repeatedly worshipped as child goddesses—but only until they have their first period ("menarche").

Jesus is undoubtedly—especially after his crucifixion—the central figure of Christianity. Initially, he was considered a Jewish itinerant preacher, later he became a prophet, and only from the Council of Nicaea (in 325) was he permanently declared a god according to the representation of the churches.

Mohammed was indeed a founder of a religion, but he never referred to himself as a god and always understood himself only as a prophet who proclaims Allah's words. He is also only revered as a prophet in Islam.

In Buddhism, Buddha is not a god—but many Buddhists often worship him as if he were a god. Or at least as an enlightened being or Bodhisattva.

8.4 God's Ground Crew

Religion was and still is an important glue of the community in many societies. In earlier times, it was like this: Besides the political authorities (princes, counts, mayors, senate, councils), the most important people of a city (or region) were doctors, judges, teachers, and **priests.** The latter had—through their (supposed) connection to the higher powers—a special role as open (or covert) advisors to the powerful. Often they were "grey eminences" who acted from the background. Some of them got carried away by this power and lost their grounding or even became megalomaniac. As a result, they had (and still have) a high power in many cultures. And for many, it was not only a highly attractive profession, but they also considered the religious activity as their vocation.

> *"All religions seem divine to the ignorant,*
> *useful to politicians*
> *and ridiculous to philosophers."*
> (Lucretius, 98–55 BC, Roman poet)

8.5 The Dilemma between Freedom and Orientation: The Vertigo of Freedom

We all have within us a tension field of two opposing needs: On the one hand, we have the desire for autonomy, freedom, independence, and self-realization. On the other hand, there is within us the need for security, for being enveloped in a meaningful, larger whole, in which we can let ourselves fall with full trust. The Danish philosopher Søren Kierkegaard called this inner conflict the "vertigo of freedom". This inner conflict accompanies us throughout our lives: Sometimes the need for autonomy and freedom is in the foreground, sometimes the need for security, comfort, and being enveloped. Basically, it is a kind of inner risk assessment: On the one hand, many young people say, "No risk, no fun." On the other hand, our knees tremble (e.g., in crises) and we long for what the psychologist of religion Sebastian Murken calls a "benevolent dependence" on credible authorities. And this is exactly where the priests and religions come into play. We are looking for trustworthy individuals and institutions that give us the feeling that everything will be fine and make sense. Tenor: There is a way out even in the most difficult situations: You will get through this crisis, you will even emerge from it stronger. This crisis is even meaningful for your personal development…

These are topics that also play an important role in many (non-religious) psychotherapy sessions. If people have had (more or less) positive experiences with religion in the course of their personal life history, these experiences can be reactivated in crises and religion can—just like psychotherapy—be helpful.

8.6 The Longing for Credible Authorities

In many myths, fairy tales, and legends, there is exactly this longing to look up to credible authorities, to admire someone who seemingly knows better and provides guidance. What manifests in secular life as a star cult (pop stars, movie stars, football greats) is in religion the mystical elevation of priests to individuals who (supposedly or only in the imagination of the believers) have a direct line to a higher being. Sometimes it is God or a saint, a bishop or even the Pope (who is often referred to as "Holy Father" and as "Vicar of God on Earth"). In other cultures, it might be a guru or Brahmin, a rabbi or mullah, a shaman or (Dalai) Lama.

What is important is that the believer considers the person in question to be credible and competent and trusts him. Then he/she is open to his support, messages, and insights. If this succeeds, it can help the believer.

8.7 Religious Authorities: Office Charisma and Personal Charisma

"Every flock needs a shepherd," was long the saying in the Catholic Church. However, not every priest is trustworthy for every believer. This always has an interpersonal relationship dimension: You can get along with one, but not with another. And of course, the framework also plays an important role. Whether the whole thing takes place in full regalia in a church setting, is it structured counseling, etc.

Is the priest present as a person and therefore credible and trustworthy? Does the fire of faith still shine from his eyes ("Who wants to shine, must burn") or does he just fulfill his church duties and simply perform his functions in his office as a priest? That's why we distinguish between **personal** and **office charisma.**

What you need to know: People who professionally deal with religions and faith—priests and theologians—are rarely objective, but almost always partisan. Since they live from it, they often represent (at least outwardly) the basic attitude and opinion of the respective institution, religious community, church or sect ("Whose bread I eat, his song I sing"). Because the task of pastors and theologians is to insert pillars of support into the house of cards of the belief system.

8.8 Enthusiastic Youth for Faith: The Exploitation of Idealism

This also includes inspiring and winning young people for faith. The recurring religious youth festivals and the Catholic World Youth Day, which takes place every three years and where the Pope usually comes and holds a mass (2023 in Lisbon), are part of this.

In earlier times, the churches did not have to advertise so much for young people, because they had (especially in rural areas) a quasi-monopoly on the exploitation of the idealism of young people. Even though it is no longer the case today: The Catholic and Protestant youth associations (including the denominational scout organizations) were the largest and most important organizations for young people in many regions.

If you go even further back in history, it was even the case that in Christian families (especially in the strictly Catholic areas) a daughter or a son had to go to the monastery—so to speak, be sacrificed to the church.

8.9 Patronizing Care

In the Catholic Church, priests are considered intermediaries between God and the faithful. To protect them from the seven deadly sins (pride, greed, lust, wrath, gluttony, envy, and sloth) and to keep the flock of believers together, priests often like to impose rules on their congregations (according to the motto "This is how you must live… this you may do—and this not"). It sometimes seems as if priests would prefer to prohibit something. Because prohibiting means: having power over someone and knowing better. Thus, there is often a very human element in the various religious communities, where pious lies and sinful holiness mix more or less elegantly. In the worst case, religious explanations of the world mix with psychotic delusion systems.

While in Hinduism there are the sacred cows that must not be slaughtered, in Islam the pigs that should not be eaten, and the dietary laws ("kosher") that are important to Jews, dietary rules play a rather minor role in Christianity. There are no fundamentally forbidden foods among Christians. At most, the prohibition of meat on Fridays among Catholics or the annual fasting period between Carnival and Easter. But these are more recommendations than commandments and prohibitions.

In contrast, the **ethical rules** from the 10 Commandments are in the foreground, some of which have found their way into our Basic Law: not lying, not stealing, no adultery, no murder and no manslaughter. The actual **religious rules** pray three times a day, Sunday service, confession after sinful behavior etc. are now only consistently incorporated into their daily lives by a few people. Most people in our latitudes have long since freed themselves from religious prescriptions.

"If you want to have an easy life,
stay with the herd."
(Friedrich Nietzsche)

The attempt to make people dependent on themselves by imposing a tight moral corset has probably failed in our region. In other regions—e.g. in southern Europe (Spain, Portugal, Italy)—it still looks different. Liberalizations are beginning there too, but a much larger part of the population still lives (at least outwardly) according to the strict Catholic norms. The violation of these norms currently mostly happens in secret. As a result, the Catholic Church (at least outwardly) still has the societal power of definition and offers a concept of salvation under its protection.

> **Heresy Objection** I have always wondered how some people have the audacity to claim they know what God wants. Whether as free-roaming prophets or as members of religious organizations.

Perhaps priests (and religious communities in general) tend to overestimate their relationship with and knowledge of God. They seriously believe they can speak to him and hear his answer. This can lead to a kind of self-overestimation. The psychoanalyst Erik Erikson writes in his Luther biography: "Luther elevated his own neurosis to that of the universal patient and then tried to solve for the world what he could not solve for himself."

> **Heresy Objection** When one speaks to God, it is called prayer. When God speaks to one—what is that? Truth? Vision? Prophecy? Or: Psychosis?

8.10 The Motivation to Become a Priest

Like many things, the choice of profession usually begins with idealism—especially when I choose a profession that has to do with religion: I want to make the world a better place, do something that advances the world for the better. This is often the motivation. Unless it is about fulfilling external expectations (e.g. in strongly religiously oriented parental homes). Which is not as rare as one often thinks.

During the course of professional training—and especially after the reality shock in the first years of the profession—not only is the idealism often lost among the young priests, but the novices are gradually conditioned to their profession and fitted into the priest role desired by the church. For some, this works well and they are satisfied with it. Others struggle with the role assigned to them and fall into intrapsychic crises. Those who struggle with it often end up in (extrachurch) psychotherapy. One patient (pastor) once told me: "We are rounded off, like a pebble on the beach." Surely this varies from person to person. Often the confessional orientation also plays an important role. Protestant priests usually have it a bit easier than Catholics. And this often has to do with celibacy.

8.11 Religions' Approach to Sexuality

Most religious communities find it difficult to deal with sexuality. It wasn't so long ago that Catholics (and in free church communities) were only allowed to have sex within marriage—and for particularly strict believers, only for the purpose of procreation. Sexual desire was considered a sin per se by many. These notions have largely been washed away by the spirit of the times.

> **Heresy Interjection** "If you want to drain a swamp, don't follow the advice of the frogs."

8.12 "Purity Culture" and "True Love Waits"

The "Purity Culture" brings back the sexually hostile basic attitude. The chastity movement "True Love Waits" (TLW) from the USA has also gained influence again in strictly Christian circles in Germany (especially in free churches outside the established religions). Sexual abstinence before marriage is propagated. The new chastity is propagated on pledge cards and through "Purity Rings" at "Purity Events".

Even though it is only a trend within a limited community, it shows the return of traditional views on sexuality.

Apart from that, in most strictly Christian communities (not only among Catholics), homosexuality is seen as sinful. Even if scoffers claim that a not insignificant part of the Catholic priests—not only in the Vatican—are homosexual.

8.13 Celibacy: Mandated Celibacy

"For some priests, it would be better,
if they were married."
(Cardinal Reinhard Marx, Spiegel 3.2.22)

Above all, the Catholic Church repeatedly comes into the public eye with the evergreen topic "Celibacy", the "celibacy" of Catholic priests mandated since the 12th century. "Eunuchs for the kingdom of heaven" is what Catholic theologian Uta Ranke-Heinemann called it. However, the sexual abstinence of priests was and is more likely the wishful thinking of the church leaders than reality.

Various studies have shown that about every second priest does not adhere to celibacy and lives in secret love relationships (with a woman or a man), and even every third priest is said to have children, who are partly even financed by the church as "children of sin"—provided the corresponding women have signed a confidentiality agreement in order not to further damage the image of the Catholic Church. Thus, hiding and lying become the basic pattern of the church, where the reputation of the church is more important than real life. It is precisely these hypocrisies, cover-ups, and sanctimonies and the compulsion for priests to lead a double life that increasingly undermine the credibility of the church organization. Some people claim that the churches are real **nurseries for neuroses**. According to the motto "We just don't talk about it", lying has been institutionalized for generations: "The holier the feast, the busier the devil."

The illusion of celibacy: The goal of celibacy is actually for the priest to not bind all his energy and love for God to one person, but to give it entirely to his congregation. Psychologically speaking, celibacy is therefore an externally mandated **repressive forced sublimation**, which not many succeed in, as most Catholic priests cannot yet deal appropriately with their unfinished sexuality. And in the worst case, this manifests itself in the sexual abuse of children and adolescents.

Klaus Kießling, Prof. Dr. theol., heads the Frankfurt Institute for Vocational Religious Education (FIBOR). He writes in the "Anzeiger für die Seelsorge" (9/2023): "However, I see a structural problem in the fact that mandatory celibacy does not necessarily have to be pathologizing in itself, but it does attract those who are already pathologized. They consciously or unconsciously associate it with the chance to conceal their own lack of ability to relate and not to have to continue dealing with their own sexuality, which has remained stuck in puberty, or even to make a virtue out of it."

Despite the discussion on the topic that has been ongoing for several years, the number of **"demerits"**, i.e., the clergy who have become criminal and who have actually been dismissed from church service and punished for their actions, is still very low.

After all the many scandals—from mass sexual abuse to various financial ambiguities and cover-ups—fewer and fewer believers trust the church leaders—throughout Central Europe. According to a study by the American PEW Research Center, in 2021/22 only 10% of the population in Germany really believe in God. In Switzerland and France, it is 11%, in the UK 12%, and in Austria, Belgium, the Czech Republic, and Estonia just 13%. And this has a lot to do with the credibility of the major churches. Because the credibility of the large faith organizations has been lost for many. Trust has been squandered. Those who preach water to the faithful and drink wine themselves are believed less and less. Who still trusts the luxury-loving aloof bishops and the various cover-up-salbadering clerics?

Meanwhile, there has been rumbling in the underground (especially) of the Catholic church communities for a long time: The faithful flock is becoming more and more insecure and rebellious. Groups like "Maria 2.0", "Church from below" and "We are Church" are putting pressure on the church leaders. Above all, the Catholic priests and bishops are irritated by the internal criticism and try to bring some calm through the "Synodal Path". Which in turn makes the Vatican clergy in Rome frown.

When I think about the sentence of my childhood pastor: "Once Catholic—always Catholic", it makes me feel quite strange. As if from baptism onwards, one can no longer escape the clutches of the church. Especially since the word meaning of Catholic is "universal, encompassing the whole".

> **Heresy Objection:**
> No, Catholicism is not dead—it just smells a bit funny.

8.14 Blasphemy: Can one blaspheme God?

*"Freedoms are not given.
Freedoms are taken."
(Aldous Huxley)*

Blasphemy refers to the insults and offenses against religious communities and/or religious confessions. However, the rejection of a religion or worldview and criticism of them are not punishable. The relevant paragraph in the penal code is § 166 StGB II. According to this, anyone who "publicly or by disseminating writings insults a church or other religious community or ideological association existing in the country, their institutions or customs in a way that is likely to disturb public peace" is liable to prosecution.

Blasphemy laws or paragraphs exist worldwide in approximately 40% of all countries (in 79 out of 198), including 14 in Europe (e.g., in Germany, Austria, Switzerland, Italy, Spain, and Finland), 12 in the Americas, 17 in Asia and Pacific states, and 18 in southern Africa (Pew Research Center, 27.07.2023). Especially in many Islamic states, blasphemy carries extremely high penalties—up to the death penalty.

> **Heresy Objection**
>
> If there is a God, one thing is certain: A real God cannot be blasphemed. He would certainly understand every position. The blasphemy paragraphs do not protect God, but at most the "ground staff of God" (i.e., priests, bishops, and popes).
>
> Blasphemies are an attack on the power positions of the church and their privileges, which—according to the view of the priests—should be unquestionable.

*"So for you, I am an atheist?
For God, I am the loyal opposition."
(Woody Allen, Stardust Memories)*

8.15 Apocalypse—or: The Pleasure in the End of the World

Since many centuries, people have occasionally assumed—partly supported by their religious beliefs—that the world is about to end. The imminent end of the world has been prophesied many hundreds of times.

With the apocalyptic sentence "The end is near", the fearful sheep are kept in the herd in many religious groups. Motto: "Only if you believe fervently and stay with us, you will be saved and live forever."

The Jehovah's Witnesses alone have already announced the end of the world several times—always with the prediction that only the 144,000 righteous will enter the post-apocalyptic heavenly kingdom (see below for more details).

The apocalypse is not a new invention: Already in the Gospel of Mark (ca. 50 AD), Jesus predicts the imminent end of the world: "Truly I tell you. There are some here who will not taste death until they see the kingdom of God coming with power." The "Revelation of John", the last book of the New Testament, also assumed an imminent apocalypse at that time.

Here is a (incomplete) selection of apocalypse ideas along historical dates:

- In the 3rd century, the followers of the Christian prophet Montanus expect the direct return of Jesus Christ and the ensuing heavenly kingdom.
- Pope Sylvester II announces that the world will end on December 31, 999. As the Christian believers fall into hysteria, Sylvester calms the congregation again by saying that his prayers have prevented the apocalypse.
- In 1532, Martin Luther announces the end of the world for the same year. When the apocalypse does not occur, he first postpones it to 1538 and then to 1541. After that, he does not commit himself anymore.
- Because of the number combination 666, which was and is considered evil, dangerous and even devilish, people also believed in the impending end of the world in 1666.
- When in 1814 the 64-year-old Miss Southcott believes she is pregnant with the new Messiah, her students and adepts assume that the world would end after the birth and only the followers would be saved. When the senior dies without giving birth to a child, her 100,000 believers interpret the situation as the child having ascended directly to heaven and would return later.
- In May 1910, Halley's comet approached the Earth. Again, mass hysteria breaks out across Europe. The believers gather in churches, confess their sins, some give away house and farm or plunge into pleasure. Several people commit suicide—out of fear of death.
- Often afterwards, lunar and solar eclipses lead to fears of the end of the world.
- As mentioned above, for Jehovah's Witnesses (JW), the year 1914 is a key date for the apocalypse. The background: The founder of JW, Charles Taze Russell, already believed in 1874 that with the year 1914 and the

beginning of World War I, the end of all earthly governments had come and finally the end of the world would come. After this, the eternal heavenly government would be established. After this did not happen, after Russell's death, his successor first announced 1916 as the year of the apocalypse, then 1918, later 1925. After JW lost a lot of members, the apocalypse was not talked about internally for a long time. Only much later, 1975 was targeted as the date of the end of the world. And after that, they do not commit themselves anymore.
- Afterwards, various sect-like organizations assume the impending end of the world: The UFO sect Aetherius Society is waiting for the extraterrestrial "Lord of Karma"—as is the St. Michael's Association. The "White Brotherhood" from Kiev even fights with the police because of this.
- The apocalypse-affine Order of the Solar Temple received special media attention because 53 members were found dead both in Switzerland and in Canada.
- In the sect "Fiat Lux", its founder Uriella assumes that everything will be over with the year 1998. She herself dies only in 2019.
- Due to the millennium change 1999/2000, many computer systems went haywire ("Millennium Bugs", "Y2K Bugs"), which in turn caused fears of the end of the world.
- In December 2012, the world was supposed to end according to the Mayan calendar.
- Etc.

Conclusion: Experienced prophets wait for the events to unfold: In retrospect, it is always easier to predict something.

References

Besier, G., Scheuch, E. K. (Eds.): Die neuen Inquisitoren Teil 1 + 2, Zürich 1999 (Edition Interfrom)
Drewermann, Eugen: Kleriker – Psychogramm eines Ideals, München 1991 (DTV)
Denzler, G. et al.: Der Ketzer Rupert Lay, Düsseldorf 1996 (Econ)
EZW Reinhard Hempelmann (Eds.): Handbuch der Evangelistisch-missionarischen Werke, Einrichtungen und Gemeinden, Stuttgart 1997 (Christliches Verlagshaus)
Esser, Wolfgang G.: Philosophische Gottsuche, München 2002 (Kösel)
Erbstösser, Martin: Ketzer im Mittelalter, Leipzig 1984 (Edition Leipzig)
Grom, Bernhard: Religionspsychologie, München 1992 (Kösel)

Ha Speis, Ralf: Spart Euch die Kirche, Würzburg 2005, 3rd edn. (KirchenOpfer)

Hempelmann, R. et al. (Eds.): Panorama der neuen Religiosität, Gütersloh 2001 (Gütersloher Verlagshaus)

Mynarek, Hubertus: Die neue Inquisition, Marktheidenfeld 1999 (Das weiße Pferd)

Mynarek, Hubertus: Herren und Knechte der Kirche, Ulm 2004 (Historia)

Niemann, U., Wagner, M.: Visionen – Werk Gottes oder Produkt des Menschen? Regensburg 2005 (Friedrich Pustet)

Schmelzer, Carsten St.: Heilung – Was wir glauben und erwarten dürfen, Witten 2013 (SCM-Brockhaus)

Schwerhoff, Gerd: Die Inquisition – Ketzerverfolgung in Mittelalter und Neuzeit, München 2004 (C.H. Beck)

Winter, Eduard: Ketzerschicksale, Düsseldorf 2002 (Albatros)

9

Levels of Religion

Summary

This chapter presents the various levels of religions and their significance: from the individual psychological level (What does religion mean for each individual believer?) to the social psychological function of religion in the immediate environment (family, reference group, circle of friends, etc.) and on the sociological level, i.e., in societal institutions (schools, associations, churches, unions, parties, etc.). It also discusses the significance of belief systems in their respective cultures and how religions have emerged throughout history. In addition, the philosophical and theological levels of religions are also presented.

*"If you want to **order the** country,
you must first put the **provinces** in order."*

*"If you want to **order the** provinces,
you must first put the **cities and villages** in order."*

*"If you want to **order the** cities and villages,
you must first put the **streets** in order."*

*"If you want to **order the** streets,
you must first put the **families** in order."*

*"If you want to **order the** families,
you must first put **your family** in order."*

*"If you want to **order your family**,
you must **order yourself** first."*
(Oriental wisdom)

Religions have various functions: They are systems of meaning for many and provide a framework of orientation: "This is right—and this is wrong." Sometimes they are the glue that holds a society together, but sometimes they also serve to exclude the "unbelievers" (In-Group—Out-Group). For some, they structure the day, for others, they create access to primal trust through certain rituals (prayers, services, meditations) and provide comfort in difficult situations.

In order to be able to judge the sense and nonsense of religions, it is necessary to look more closely at the various levels at which they are effective, to differentiate and analyze them.

The following levels of religion can be distinguished:

1. Theological level
2. Philosophical/ethical level
3. Historical and cultural level
4. Sociological level
5. Social psychological level
6. Individual psychological level

9.1 Theological Level

The theological level is something like the core competence of each religion: Here you will find the specific beliefs:

What exactly should/may/must I believe? What is the internal image of God within the religion? Which belief system should I follow? What are the rules and prohibitions? What holy books are there? What are the unquestionable dogmas? What rituals, prayers, meditations, services are required? How strictly must the duties be adhered to? Are there sanctions for non-compliance? How should faith be lived in everyday life? What are the rules for a "God-pleasing life"?

These questions of faith differ quite significantly among the individual religious groups. Not only between Christians and Muslims, Jews and Buddhists, Hindus and Taoists—but also within the major religious directions: Catholics argue with Protestants. And within the Protestants, the Lutherans argue with the Reformed. And within the Reformed, the Calvinists and the Hussites argue…

9.2 Philosophical Level

"The difference between religion and philosophy is, that philosophy assumes the equivalence of good and evil."

On the philosophical level, it is generally about values, ethics, and morals. Concepts such as love, compassion, responsibility, trust, and loyalty play a role, as do solidarity, security, justice, honesty, commitment, courage, or reliability, respect, honor, reverence, tolerance, and (self-)discipline.

These values are not inherently related to religions. They not only play a role in religions but are also found in atheistic or agnostic worldviews. The values of the French Revolution (liberty, equality, fraternity) also belong to philosophical topics.

9.3 Historical and Cultural Level

Did cultures arise from religion—or did religion arise from cultures? This is like the question: Which came first, the chicken or the egg? Religion and culture have developed simultaneously and have influenced and shaped each other—and continue to do so to this day. The differences between a Christian-influenced culture and an Islamic or Buddhist one can be significant and may be further amplified by the religions.

Since changes in cultures are slow and happen slowly, they take their time. However, religions, with their statically oriented dogmas, are usually the ones that slow down change processes. This can be exemplified by the current changes in gender roles in Western countries: The discussion about hetero-, queer-, bi-, non-binary-, pansexuality, or gender fluidity is a thorn in the side of most religiously oriented people—whether strictly Catholic, Orthodox, Jewish, or Islamic—because they usually assume a clear and exclusive binary gender, which they find in their holy books: There is only either man or woman. This position must not be questioned. This attitude points to the general problem of dogmatism. As long as the dogmatists believe "Only we are right", this will not change. It is an attempt to adapt the landscape to the map—not the other way around.

9.4 Sociological Level

We live in a time when *weak* social ties are increasing, but *strong* ties are decreasing. This is evident, for example, in online acquaintances: What does it mean if you have 200 friends on Facebook? Will they be able to help me in a real crisis?

Mobility and flexibility have become almost obligatory for many—especially young people—(especially if they want to be successful in their careers): Many follow their jobs. And usually towards big cities—simply because there are often better professional positions there. More and more (especially young) people are moving from small communities (where they may still have had sufficient social contacts) to big cities—and thus into anonymity and possibly into loneliness. It sometimes takes a lot of effort to constantly build up a new circle of friends—if it succeeds at all.

This is accompanied by a gradual departure from traditional family life. The divorce rate is extremely high (almost 40%)—as is the number of single households: 41% (2021). In addition to traditional father-mother families and single parents, there is now a veritable "love**dis**order" with a variety of different couple and family forms:

- LAT: Living apart together (separate cohabitation)
- DINKs: Double income no kids (double income, no children)
- DCCs: Dual career couples (career couples)
- "Patchwork families"
- Etc.

And this is happening against increasingly fragile psychological structures (so-called "patchwork identities") and of course has an influence on attitudes towards religion. The church's views on the following topics are increasingly less in demand:

- Finding meaning (and thus religiosity) is no longer automatically socially predetermined, but must be sought individually.
- There is less and less religious education: new socialization conditions.
- The "blinding power" of religions has dramatically decreased.
- The social pressure to be a member of a religious community has greatly decreased: Everyone can and should be happy in their own way—with whatever belief system.

- The pressure to be individual, on the other hand, has increased significantly: One must show oneself as a person, performance must be delivered personally, etc.
- Personal style: From nothing by chance to individuality?
- New norms of life practice: Men's and women's roles have changed, gender role diffusion (not only) in children and adolescents.
- Changed relationship patterns in friendships, partnerships, and marriages (from monogamy to polygamy to polyamory).
- Dealing with sexuality: Heterosexuality, homosexuality, bi-sexuality etc. Forms of contraception: Condom, coil, pill, abortion etc.
- Other family forms: Patchwork families, single-parent family, sequential monogamy, chain marriages, parenting issues, etc.

9.5 Social Psychological Level

On the social psychological level, the concrete, direct, social living environment is in the foreground. Life in the community, in the family, and in the circle of friends. It's about social support—but possibly also about social control. In relation to religious communities: How often am I in the church or the church community? Do I regularly attend spiritual events? Is there perhaps something like a home circle or prayer circle? What religious rituals are practiced there: Services, communion, confession, yoga, satsang, dhikr … Are there recurring consecrations of people, objects, places, canonizations etc. in the direct environment?

9.6 Individual Psychological Level

Here it is about the individual psychological processing of one's own religiosity:

- What is happening on my inner stage? What does my faith mean to me? How important are my personal values to me? To what extent do I really live by them?
- Do I have real intrapsychic help through this? Do I really develop something like "basic trust" through my faith? Do I feel arrived and accepted in the world? Is there something like a certainty of faith for me?
- How important was (and is) religious support for me in times of change and crisis?

- What significance do the spiritual transition or passage rites have for me: Baptism, Communion, Confession, Confirmation, Confirmation, Marriage, Last Rites etc.
- Does the mystical dimension in religions play a role for me? Is it positively charged or does it scare me?
- Have I already had spiritual-mystical experiences myself?
- Does religion have an influence on my everyday life design?

References

Esser, Wolfgang G.: Philosophische Gottsuche, München 2002 (Kösel)
Kolbe, Christoph: Heilung oder Hindernis – Religion bei Freud, Adler, Fromm, Jung und Frankl, Stuttgart 1986 (Kreuz)
Metz, Wulf (Eds.): Handbuch Weltreligionen, Wuppertal 2003 (Brockhaus)
Schnabel, Ulrich: Die Vermessung des Glaubens, München 2008 (Blessing)
Volf, Miroslav: Zusammen wachsen – Globalisierung braucht Religion, Gütersloh 2017 (Gütersloher Verlagshaus)

Left

Das säkulare Jahrzehnt: Wie sich Deutschland verändern wird – YouTube (Stand: 16.8.2023)

Part III

The External and Internal Aspects of Religions

10

Religious Organizations: From the Faith Community to the Sect to the Church

> **Summary**
>
> This chapter deals with the societal role of religious organizations: Churches, Sects and religious faith communities of all kinds. What are the commonalities of church groups and where are the differences? When and how are they helpful and where do they become problematic or even dangerous? Are they part of the problem or part of the solution? Where are they the bridge of believers to their God and what about their power? How do they gain significance for the individual member and what role do they play in society?

*"Whoever believes to be a Christian,
because he attends church, is mistaken.
You don't become a car,
just by going into a garage."*
(Albert Schweitzer)

The two major churches are powerful institutions in our country. They accompany us from the cradle to the grave. From contraception and baptism to euthanasia, they are involved in many things. In the field of education, they run kindergartens, schools, and universities. They are involved in the stages of life with communion and confirmation. They try to influence sexual behavior, are involved in (church) marriage as well as in hospital pastoral care and the last anointing. Churches feel responsible for everything—but are they also accountable? Undoubtedly, habits and traditions are important for people, and religious rules provide orientation, but they are also restrictions: What is right, what is wrong? And the question is: Who still adheres to them? Not least for this reason, the two major churches try to bring these topics to people in bite-sized pieces:

"Finally living" was the title of the program booklet of the Catholic House at the Cathedral (Frankfurt) at the beginning of 2023. The organizers were concerned with the ambiguity of this term. On the one hand: "So-now-finally-start-with-the-good-life", on the other hand, a look should also be taken at the finiteness of human existence. The individual human life is not infinite: When do I really live? What do I do with my lifetime? What is the purpose of my life?

What is often forgotten: Both churches are huge economic enterprises. They are not only land, forest, and real estate owners, but they also own a lot of companies or are involved in them. The total business of the two churches has a volume of about 130 billion €. And they are among the largest employers in Germany. Together they have about 1.8 million employees—of which about 1.3 million are in the two major welfare associations Diakonie (Protestant) and Caritas (Catholic). In addition, they collected about 13 billion € in church taxes in 2022 (Catholic Church: 6.8 billion, Protestant Church: 6.1 billion).

10.1 The Societal Role of Religious Communities

"Religion is that,
which prevents the poor from,
killing the rich."
(Napoleon)

People and groups of people set rules for themselves and like to invoke God/gods to make them unassailable and irrevocable. Religious communities often use this approach to present these rules as "god-given" and not open to question. Especially when they already had a certain power in a social group and access to the respective elites, they could influence or even determine the rules of conduct. Because the missionary aspect was and is always important to religious communities, i.e., to enforce their faith and their point of view.

If one looks at the historical dimension of the churches, one can see how much the individual religions have adopted from each other. Not only were the temples and churches of the new faith built on the ruins of the previous religions, but holidays and rituals were also copied or modified.

> *"Good tradition*
> *is the passing on of the fire*
> *– not the worship of the ashes."*
> *(Gustav Mahler)*

For Christians, it was a long journey from the small persecuted, sect-like religious community in ancient Rome to the power structure that is capable of influencing, regulating, and controlling entire nations at the political level.

The major churches have usually conspired with the powerful from an early stage. Emperors, kings, tsars, princes, and counts had church advisors—sometimes they were even the secret rulers, who as black-gray eminences covertly had the say. And this did not always happen for the benefit of the entire population.

From the old emperors in the early Middle Ages to the present day, they have established themselves in many forms of government. And also in many authoritarian systems, various religious organizations have allowed themselves to be made the whore of politics and have provided legitimations for all kinds of atrocities.

10.2 Religious Flags in the Wind

In the monarchy they were monarchists, in democracy they were democratic, in fascism they were fascist—in the Nazi era sometimes racist. At Christmas and Easter, they often speak of peace, but they also like to bless war weapons (most recently the Orthodox Church in the Ukraine war).

You can call this "adapted realpolitik" or "spiritual flexibility"—or opportunism for the preservation of power—no matter who is in charge.

An old heretic saying goes:

> *"'Keep them stupid',*
> *said the prince to the bishop,*
> *'I'll keep them poor'."*

And throughout history, priests have been involved in many inhumane processes and systems: In addition to the persecution of Jews and the burning of witches, they also legitimized slavery in the USA. Pope Pius XII conspired with Hitler in the Concordat, while the Protestants offered themselves antisemitically to Hitler as "German Christians" and demanded "racial purity".

Whether it was about supporting the fascist Franco regime in Spain or Salazar in Portugal and Pinochet in Chile—the churches were always dealing with the powerful. Even the former apartheid regime in South Africa could once enjoy church support.

> **Heretic interjection** Religious organizations are not inherently corrupt or criminal—but they can easily become so …

10.3 Counter-movements within the Church

Fairly it must be said, however, that there have always been counter-movements within the churches against the collusion with the powerful—e.g. the "Confessing Church", which resisted Nazi conformity. Or Nelson Mandela and Bishop Tutu, who helped overcome apartheid. Not to underestimate—in overcoming the authoritarian communist regime in Poland, the Catholic Church played an important role by supporting Lech Walesa. Also worth mentioning are the South American liberation theologians around the murdered Archbishop Romero, who developed as a counterpoint to the conservative established Catholics.

Thus, at all times and in many regions, there are almost always various grassroots movements that resist the unhealthy entanglements with the powerful.

10.4 The Limited Tolerance of Religions

Religions are usually tolerant only as long as they are not in power. When they have the opportunity to restrict or hinder other belief systems, they often do so. The goal is almost always to attribute the grace of salvation exclusively to their own faith.

After all, "Catholic" means "universal". So when the Pope, as Pontifex Maximus (high priest), proclaims that only Catholics can achieve grace and salvation, this has a centuries-old tradition. Already in the year 250 AD, the Church Father Cyprian of Carthage proclaimed: "Extra ecclesiam salus non est" ("Outside the Church there is no salvation").

10.5 The Infallibility of the Pope

The **1st Vatican Council** declared on July 18, 1870, that the Pope, when he speaks "ex cathedra" and as God's representative on earth, is **infallible**: "The holy Mother Church holds and teaches that God, the origin and goal of all things, can certainly be recognized by the natural light of human reason from the created things" (Dei Filius DS 3004). In addition, at the same council, Pius IX condemned freedom of belief and opinion, as well as the separation of church and state.

10.6 Religious Communities: Freedom and Democracy

Religious organizations are rarely truly democratic, because the belief system is almost always more important than democracy. Some, however, occasionally adopt a democratic facade (e.g., in church council elections, church board elections). But the believers are not really allowed to have a say in the correct or incorrect faith.

And freedom movements and democratic aspirations were usually rather suspect or even an abomination to the servants of God. Insurgent peasants and workers were considered godless because they questioned the rule(s) of the powerful.

Even Martin Luther, who had rebelled against the authority of the Catholic Church and fought against it, wrote in 1525 the treatise "Against the Murderous and Thieving Hordes of Peasants", in which he called on the princely rulers in the war to kill the revolting peasants, praising this as religiously meritorious deeds.

10.7 Churches and Sects

There are more similarities between churches and sects than the established churches want to admit. Both are faith and religious communities. While "church" is a self-designation, "sect" is a fighting term used to try to discredit others.

After all, almost all of them started as a sect—namely as a split-off. Something about the traditional religion did not suit them and they found and spread the "true faith" for them. And this in contrast to the traditional and conventional religion. Thus, one could say that the early Christians were actually a Jewish sect. When comparing the various religions, the differences and rivalries are usually in the foreground.

10.8 Project World Ethos

But there are also counter-movements that try to emphasize not the differences, but the commonalities between the various (world) religions.

This includes above all the "Project World Ethos", which the former Catholic priest and theology professor Hans Küng initiated in the early 1990s. His goal was to establish the common ethics of the world religions as a minimal basic consensus with unalterable standards and moral attitudes.

This involves general values such as humanity, justice, truthfulness, non-violence, equal partnership, and ecological responsibility. These principles are laid down in the "Declaration of the World Ethos", which was adopted in Chicago in 1993 under Küng's leadership by several hundred representatives of religions. Hans Küng was considered one of the most prominent church critics in the German-speaking world, who was particularly opposed to the dogma of papal infallibility—which is why he was deprived of his ecclesiastical teaching authority in 1979. Küng was president of the World Ethos Foundation, which he co-founded, until 2013. He died on April 6, 2021.

The still existing World Ethos Foundation continues to advocate for the above-mentioned values, but is rather only touched with kid gloves by the major churches.

10.9 Caricature and Enemy Image

There is a caricature and an enemy image of virtually every religion. The question is how much one feeds this enemy image or maintains an objective view of the respective faith. Sometimes, however, reality in its strangeness even surpasses the caricature. Even parts of American hard-core Christianity, which is loudly and hucksterishly proclaimed by its sometimes megalomaniac preachers and "prophets", try with their magical-sectarian understanding of faith, sometimes even to push dear God through prayers, so that he finally does what they wish. Fortunately, God cannot be bribed by prayers or services, but it is usually only a coincidence if something succeeds.

Despite the Christian vows of poverty, obedience, and chastity, the issue of money plays a central role, especially in the circles of religious US prophets. After all, the huge church-like glass palaces, the internet appearances, and the opulent lifestyle of the preachers also need to be financed—where "money laundering with holy water" apparently is not uncommon.

10.10 Religion on the Internet

In today's times, however, one must say: Anyone can nowadays try to introduce a new belief system on the internet or even found a new religion. And even the most extreme new religious belief theory finds a few followers somewhere in the world in internet times. Even the most twisted sect guru has at least one adept—otherwise, he would probably end up in psychiatry.

And there is an almost unmanageable amount of different belief systems circulating and being propagated on the internet. And each considers their ideas to be the final plan for saving the world.

> *"Idiots are a wise arrangement of nature.*
> *They allow fools to think they are smart."*
> *(George Bernard Shaw)*

What one must not forget in all the criticism of religious communities: There is nothing to say against the true core of religions—namely developing basic trust, giving hope, without creating illusions. The problems begin with the dogmas of faith of the individual religious systems, namely when one clings so firmly to one's own truth and considers it the only correct and eternally true one and devalues or fights all others.

References

Bernhardt, Reinhold: Der Absolutheitsanspruch des Christentums, Gütersloh 1990 (Gütersloher Verlagshaus)

Bartel, Karlheinz: Meditation – was ist das? Stuttgart 1996 (Kreuz)

Bork, Uwe: Kleines Lexikon biblischer Irrtümer, Gütersloh 2009 (Gütersloher Verlagshaus)

Denzler, G. et al.: Der Ketzer Rupert Lay, Düsseldorf 1996 (Econ)

Feldtkeller, Andreas: Warum denn Religion? Gütersloh 2006 (Gütersloher Verlagshaus)

Gross, Werner: Wie man lebt, so stirbt man, Berlin/Heidelberg 2021 (Springer)
Gross, Werner: Was Sie schon immer über Sucht wissen wollten, Berlin/Heidelberg 2016 (Springer)
Holl, Adolf: Im Keller des Heiligtums, Stuttgart 1991 (Kreuz)
Linke, Detlef B.: Religion als Risiko – Geist, Glaube und Gehirn, Reinbek 2005 (Rowohlt)
Poppelreuter, S; Gross, W. (Hrsg).: Nicht nur Drogen machen süchtig, Weinheim 2000 (PVU)
Speis, Ralf: Spart Euch die Kirche, Würzburg 2005, 3. Aufl. (KirchenOpfer)
Tempelmann, Inge: Geistlicher Missbrauch – Auswege aus frommer Gewalt, Wuppertal 2007 (Brockhaus)
Weidinger, Erich: Die Apokryphen – Verborgene Bücher der Bibel, Augsburg 1994 (Pattloch)
Zander, Hans Conrad: Kurzgefasste Verteidigung der Heiligen Inquisition, Gütersloh 2007 (Gütersloher Verlagshaus)

Left

Kirchenaustritt.de

11

Religious Enlightenment Experiences and Altered States of Consciousness

> **Summary**
>
> This chapter focuses on the intrapsychic processing of mystical-religious experiences. What happens in a person when someone has an "enlightenment experience"—physically, neurologically, psychologically? What happens when someone falls into a "spiritual crisis"? What leads to a "metanoia", a reversal of inner values?

"I didn't know what I was looking for, before I found it."

11.1 "Homo Religiosus": Numinous Experiences

Serious religiosity has to do with the innermost core of a person, which is to a considerable extent unconscious. But there is a generalized metaphysical dissatisfaction and a need for transcendence and mystical elevation of life in many spiritual people. They seek to transcend boundaries, want to grow beyond themselves and merge with the world and the cosmos. For a considerable number of these people, something like "enlightenment" is an important goal of personality development: "egolessness", "merging with the primal ground of being", "connection with the primal force of life" are descriptive terms for inner experiences that are difficult to put into words.

In Zen Buddhism, one speaks of "Satori" (enlightenment, understanding) or "Nirvana", the extinction of desires and ignorance and thus exit from the cycle of suffering, the so-called "wheel of rebirths" (Samsara). In Hinduism, the desired state is called "Moksha" (salvation). In Jewish Kabbalism, it is called "En-Sof", the unspeakable, the infinite.

In Christianity, it is perhaps called "God experience" or "holy spirit". Often, those affected are fascinated by all things numinous(mysterious, inexplicable). Behind this often lies the desire to understand the incomprehensible, and also the longing to be initiated into the mysteries of life. But this is easier said than done. For only when one is also inwardly mature and ready, will one have the corresponding experiences.

"The mystery protects itself," is a key sentence of the old mystics, which means that only the person who is mature and able to understand what is happening to them, will consciously have this experience. And above all, draw the right conclusions from it to change their life in the right way ("metanoia"). This is supposed to be a foretaste of eternity and immortality, the eternal now.

"You only understand it if you have experienced it yourself," it is said in mysticism.

For religious experiences are subjective truths, which are to be appreciated and respected. Consider: "When you have access to the innermost of a person, you are entering holy ground."

These intense states of experience and feeling are difficult to put into words because they are highly subjective. "The small truth has many words. The great truth has only silence," say the Zen Buddhists.

11.2 Enlightenment in a Crash Course: "Illuminatio præcox"

Thesemystical experiences, possibly gained through long-term religious practices, are contrasted with spontaneous enlightenment experiences that happen to some people out of nowhere (or were provoked by spiritual exercises) and are sometimes difficult to understand and integrate into the mental state.

"Enlightenment doesn't care how you achieve it" was the title of a small book by Thaddeus Golas in the 1980s, which has achieved a certain cult status in the spiritual scene. And it also addressed the hunger for miracles, madness, and dissolution: On the psycho-market and in the esoteric scene, there are plenty of methods and techniques used to provoke these enlightenment experiences. Situations are heavily charged with meaning to enable intense experiences. The range extends from the use of psychoactive substances (LSD, mescaline, ecstasy, ayahuasca …) to certain spiritual methods (excessive prayer and meditation, chanting) and cathartic body psychotherapeutic techniques (ecstasy and trance dances, bioenergetics, rebirthing, primal scream, etc.) to drastic interventions in everyday life (sleep deprivation, fasting, sensory deprivation).

> *"If you don't understand, a tree is a tree."*
> *"When you start to understand, the tree is no longer a tree."*
> *"When you have understood, a tree is (again) a tree."*
> (Zen)

However: Those who seek the highest are also at risk of falling deeply: "Whoever climbs higher than he should, falls (if he is not careful) deeper than he wanted."

Undoubtedly, some people have intense, partly also positive, boundary experiences in a weekend crash course—but unfortunately, it happens all too often that people are thrown off track by this and come home confused because they cannot understand and integrate what they have experienced. In the worst case, someone decompensates through these experiences and ends up in psychiatry due to a psychotic episode. Because the wall between enlightenment and delusion is sometimes wafer-thin. Thus, enlightenment can also become a horror trip that changes life in a completely wrong direction. All you can say is: "Be careful with enlightenment."

> **Heretical Interjection** How many enlightenment experiences are the offspring of an extended seed madness?

Excursus: What is Mysticism?

> **Mysticism**
>
> The term "mystical" is often used in everyday language to mean "mysterious", "incomprehensible" or "enigmatic". However, there is a mystical dimension in all religions. The goal of mysticism is the unification with a higher power, an energy, or the immersion in God. Religious externals (rituals, prayers, services, dogmas, etc.) are secondary, as they are used at best as tools to achieve the mystical state. Often, the dogmas are experienced by the mystic as a constraint from which he seeks to free himself. Some mystics are therefore persecuted as heretics (not only in Christianity), but some are also declared saints (see below).

> In Christianity, Meister Eckhart, Johannes Tauler, Teresa of Avila, Hildegard of Bingen, Ignatius of Loyola, Francis of Assisi, etc. are known as mystics.
> The mystic is concerned with his very subjective-personal relationship to his God ("unio mystica"). The mystical path is emotional and experience-oriented. Sometimes ecstatic ("happiness") experiences ("expansion of consciousness", "breakthrough into another reality", "enlightenment") are sought and reported. These experiences are usually very intense, but rather short-lived. Mystical experiences are all-encompassing and paradoxical. They are intuitive and often associated with an "oceanic feeling". The tenor is: "Everything is one." It is difficult to put mystical experiences into words. Lao-Tse says: "Those who say it, do not know it. Those who know it, do not say it." In the Christian area, it would be called "silentium mysticum". However, it is not easy to develop a mystical lifestyle from this intense faith experience.

11.3 Mystical Traditions

"Stand firm in this world -
and only then lean towards the other."
(Mystic Wisdom)

There is a mystical dimension and tradition in virtually all religions. Normally, mystics of all religious traditions understand each other quite well across religious boundaries. Whether it's Islamic Sufis, Buddhist monks, Christian mystics, Jewish Hasidim, or Rosicrucians and Freemasons, they seem to have "tuned in" to a common—mystical—wavelength.

Mysticism can be understood as the self-emptying search for higher realities, for transcendence ("ecstasy") and intense spiritual experiences. Mystics are concerned with unification, merging with, and dissolving into a higher being. This can be nature or God.

"Whoever has God,
to him all things taste of God."
(Meister Eckhart)

Augustine had already written in his text "On True Religion": "Do not go outside. Retreat into yourself. Truth dwells within."

Meister Eckhart (1260–1327) also believed that God could be found in all things. Although one does not see him directly, for him, God is everywhere. And he taught that a separation of God and the world is an illusion.

This was too far for the Church and was condemned as heresy by Pope John XXII in a papal bull.

And so it went (and continues to this day) with almost all mystical traditions: First they are welcomed as a renewal and revival of faith: "Do not worship the ashes, but kindle the fire of faith in you." Because mystics are actually anarchists and do not adhere to the prescribed norms and religious rules, they are usually first pushed to the margins, later ostracized and banned, and eventually perhaps even persecuted. This applies to the Sufis in Islam as well as to the Christian mystics (Meister Eckhart, Hildegard of Bingen, Johannes Tauler, Jakob Böhme …). They are then often declared heretics—and a few generations later they are rediscovered to renew faith again …

11.4 Unio Mystica: Union with God

"Die before you die."
(Sufism)

A mystic might say something like this about themselves:

"If I manage to ally myself so intensely with God, then I feel one with an infinitely strong, unlimited power. This can lead to the feeling that I can achieve anything (with God's help)—because nothing is impossible for God, nothing is impossible for me. I feel merged with him, I am his executing organ, his tool."

This can sound like psychotic "delusions of grandeur", as the mystic naturally also relinquishes his responsibility to a (diffuse, but very concrete inner) power. However, there are a multitude of dangers on the path to enlightenment that the adept must overcome. In the Bahai, the smallest and youngest world religion, they speak of the "Seven Valleys" that a true believer should traverse:

1. The Valley of Seeking
2. The Valley of Love
3. The Valley of Knowledge
4. The Valley of Unity
5. The Valley of Contentment
6. The Valley of Wonderment
7. The Valley of True Poverty and Absolute Nothingness

Because this journey (the Sufis call it the "path") is so full of stumbling blocks, most traditional mystical paths also have a strict master-student relationship. Since the long-standing masters know and have overcome the dangers of the mystical path (should have), they are guides and companions of the mystic adept. This naturally also involves a close and dependent relationship of the student with his master. This can push the issue of authority to the forefront until the student is ready to go his own way.

In Buddhism it is said: "If you meet Buddha on the road—kill him." This is not a call to murder, but means that the adept should accept no one more than Buddha (i.e., as a kind of saintly figure). But despite this independence, the mystic remains part of the traditional line, which the Sufis call "chain".

11.5 The Mystery of Consciousness

Even though there is no universally valid definition of consciousness to this day, it can be said that these spiritual experiences almost always happen in an altered state of consciousness.

From various studies, we know that adults spend about 60% of their time in a waking state, about 12% in deep sleep, 10% in light sleep, and 8% in dream sleep. The remaining approximately 10% is then left for daydreams, sub-trances, and altered states of consciousness, which in highly spiritual people are often filled with religious content (e.g., seeking God). It is important to realize that all experiences are interpreted experiences. And many religious experiences are often illusions experienced as true: They consist—in short—of perception and interpretation of perception.

"Serious spirituality
can be divided into twelve areas,
eleven parts silence,
one part speaking cautiously and quietly."
(Mystic Wisdom)

Heretical Objection Is prayer more than a form of autosuggestion, self-hypnosis, and magical practice?

11.6 Altered States of Consciousness and Enlightenment Experiences

"Meditating is still better than sitting around doing nothing."

Religiousexperiences are not only manifested in conscious experience, but are intense emotional experiences that are also neurologically detectable in the limbic system.

One thing is certain: God only finds one way into our heads—namely through the nerve pathways of our brain. Because altered states of consciousness are associated with strong positive feelings, such as ecstasy, intoxication, and pleasurable feelings of boundary dissolution. However, they can also evoke intense feelings of fear and loss of control: enlightenment can also be experienced as a kind of mental catastrophe.

These conditions are also called extraordinary states of consciousness (ESC). They are usually characterized by the following characteristics:

- Clearly detectable deviations of subjective experience and/or mental functioning from waking consciousness, self-forgetfulness.
- Sensory consciousness changes: Enhanced sensory perceptions, synaesthesia (seeing sounds, tasting colors).
- Change in cognition and thinking, mood and motor activity, overall self-consciousness.
- Loss of control (partly positively pleasurable, partly associated with intense fear).
- Unusual environmental experience—spatial grid can change: In subjective perception, walls bend, ceilings bulge, near-far distance shifts.
- The sense of time changes: Seconds seem eternally long, hours accelerate or shorten in perception.
- The person experiences themselves as "strange", "funny", "abnormal".
- Changes in body schema can occur. Situations are experienced as irrational, exotic, pathological. Sometimes: psychosis-like and fear-inducing ("enlightenment delirium").
- But there can also be dramatic positive experiences: feelings of happiness, unity of inner and outer world, becoming one with God, the higher self or nature, near-death experiences etc.
- Mobilization of the inner self-healing powers: "Miracle healings" in trance are possible.

Such a state can be short-term (seconds or minutes). But it can also last for hours.

Adolf Dittrich described the following altered states of consciousness in 1996 and categorized them as follows:

1. **Oceanic self-dissolution (OSE):** Positive feelings, no separation of inside and outside, connection with the cosmos, pleasurable loss of control, primary-narcissistic sensations
2. **Fearful ego dissolution (AIA):** Negative tone, problematic loss of control, fear up to panic attack
3. **Visionary restructuring (VUS):** Depending on how much of the experienced can be implemented in everyday life

In general, one can say: These are always experiences of boundary dissolution, mental exceptional states, which can be positive (fulfilling, nourishing, trust-building), but also problematic (fear- or panic-inducing, "horror trip"): When the angels show themselves, the devils are usually not far away.

11.7 Triggers of Extraordinary States of Consciousness

Different triggers of extraordinary states of consciousness can be distinguished.

11.8 Chemical and Pharmacological Triggers

Extraordinary states of consciousness can be triggered by chemical and pharmacological drugs (not uncommon in the esoteric scene):

- First order hallucinogens (LSD, mescaline, psilocybin etc.)
- Second order hallucinogens (nitrous oxide, muscimol, scopolamine etc.)
- Various other psychedelics

When the drug is present, its use is usually quite simple and effortless. The effect is quick and intense. However, there is a high risk of addiction not to be underestimated (not to mention the side effects that can be caused by adulterants in illegal drugs).

11.9 Psychological Triggers

Through certain behaviors and circumstances, extraordinary states of consciousness can also be produced without the use of drugs:

- Reduction of environmental stimulation or contact (sensory deprivation, meditation, AT, hypnosis etc.)
- Overstimulation, monotonous rhythmic stimulation, overexertion (physical and psychological, fear-pleasure mobilization)
- Destabilization (sleep deprivation, fasting, dehydration, hypoglycemia, hyperventilation etc.)

The psychological triggers require effort, take longer and are less intense, but they also rarely have lasting physical side effects.

These techniques are often used in religions and in the esoteric scene to provoke spiritual experiences ("conversion", "transformation" "experiencing God").

11.10 "God Helmet": Electromagnetic Triggers of Spiritual Feelings?

The "God Helmet" is a modified motorcycle helmet that exposes the human brain (specifically the temporal lobe region) to a small magnetic field. This stimulation of the magnetic field is supposed to be able to generate spiritual feelings. According to Canadian psychology professor Michael Persinger, this transcranial magnetic stimulator was able to induce religious experiences in 80% of all subjects (e.g., the presence of a higher being, experiences of God, encounters with angels). Persinger assumed that the God Helmet in transcranial magnetic stimulation (TMS) would cause micro-seizures of temporal lobe epilepsy, which many subjects would interpret as religiosity ("God Concept"). For several subjects, this seemed to have worked, but others simply felt sick. And still others became only anxious or angry.

11.11 Does God Live in the Brain?

So can religious experiences be induced by means of TMS? What then is the value of religion—if God perhaps only lives in the brain? Or if God is perhaps just a figment of the brain? Since these experiments caused a loud noise in the media forest and produced intense, sometimes panic-like reactions among priests and theologians, because it would have shaken various religious foundations, efforts were made to quickly counteract this.

Psychologist Pehr Granqvist at the Swedish University of Uppsala was unable to verify this experiment in a double-blind study. Many subjects in the control group, whose helmet had not been activated at all, also reported religious experiences (placebo effect). Other attempts at reproduction also failed.

11.12 "God Module"

Indian neuroscientist and brain researcher Vilaynur S. Ramachandran at the University of San Diego, however, did not rule out that divine appearances could be produced by appropriate temporal lobe stimulation. He assumed that the fundamentally higher-oriented neuronal circuits in connection with the overload of unprocessed experiences were a kind of "God Module" that could be activated by TMS. In his investigations, he made no distinction whether it was Buddhist monks or Catholic nuns. Whether Christianity, Islam or Hinduism—religiosity takes place in the same brain area for all religions.

Within the "scientific community", however, the approaches of Ramachandran and Persinger are not considered particularly serious.

11.13 Neurotheology

Nevertheless, Ramachandran's investigations—in addition to the older findings of Persinger and various studies on the use of psilocybin—were the foundation of "Neurotheology". This is a scientific approach that aims to investigate religious-spiritual experiences with methods of neurobiology.

11.14 Conclusion

What do all the scientific findings tell us? One thing is certain: All our experiences, including religious ones, are perceived, processed, and stored in the brain. But does that make God a figment of the imagination? God cannot be scientifically proven, that's for sure. However, it also cannot be scientifically proven that he does not exist.

*"Do not grow weary,
but to the miracle,
quiet as a bird,
extend your hand."
(Hilde Domin)*

References

Bucher, Anton A.: Psychologie der Spiritualität, Weinheim 2007 (Beltz)

Blume, M. und Vaas, R.: Gott, Gene und Gehirn. Warum Glaube nützt. Die Evolution der Religiosität Stuttgart 2022 (Hirzel)

Bartel, Karlheinz: Meditation—was ist das?, Stuttgart 1996 (Kreuz)

Bragdon, Emma: Spirituelle Krisen—Wendepunkte im Leben, Freiburg 1991 (Bauer)

Collins, Francis S.: Gott und die Gene, Gütersloh 2007 (Gütersloher Verlagshaus)

Eibach, Ulrich: Gott im Gehirn? Ich—eine Illusion?, Wuppertal 2006 (R. Brockhaus)

Hamer, Dean: Das Gottes-Gen, München 2006 (Kösel)

Harris, Marvin: Fauler Zauber—unsere Sehnsucht nach der anderen Welt, Stuttgart 1993 (Klett-Cotta)

Hoffmann, Ulrich: Was Meditation wirklich kann, München 2018 (O.W. Barth)

Hochstrasser, Josef: Religion ist heilbar, Basel 2007 (Zytglogge)

James, William: Die Vielfalt religiöser Erfahrung, Olten 1979 (Walter)

Linke, Detlef B.: Religion als Risiko—Geist, Glaube und Gehirn, Reinbek 2005 (Rowohlt)

Linnewedel, Jürgen: Mystik—Meditation—Yoga—Zen, Stuttgart 1975 (Quell)

Maezumi Roshi, T., Glassmann Roshi, B. T.: Erleuchtung—was ist das?, München 2002 (O.W. Barth)

Milzner, Georg: Religion und Gehirn—Die Integration von Hirnforschung und religiöser Erfahrung, Petersberg 2013 (Via Nova)

Mönter, Norbert (Hrsg.): Seelische Erkrankung, Religion und Sinndeutung, Bonn 2007 (Psychiatrie-V.)

Meister Eckehart: Deutsche Predigten und Traktate, München 1963 (Hanser)

Niemann, U., Wagner, M.: Visionen—Werk Gottes oder Produkt des Menschen?, Regensburg 2005 (Friedrich Pustet)

Noort, Tamar: Die Ewigkeit ist ein guter Ort, Reinbek 2022 (Rowohlt)

Schweid, Richard: Sehnsucht nach Unsterblichkeit, Gütersloh 2008 (Gütersloher Verlagshaus)

Scharfetter, Christian: Der spirituelle Weg und seine Gefahren, Stuttgart 1999 (Thieme)

Schmelzer, Carsten St.: Heilung—Was wir glauben und erwarten dürfen, Witten 2013 (SCM-Brockhaus)

Left

Gotteshelm | Drogen Wiki | Fandom (Stand: 19.9.2023)
Neurotheologie—Wikipedia (Stand: 19.9.2023)

12

What is Sacred to Me—or: Blessing is the Ability to Give Something You Don't Have Yourself

> **Summary**
>
> This chapter addresses the question of what is actually sacred. Is there "the sacred" as an objective fact—for example, sacred places, sacred rituals, sacred people? Or is sacred always just a subjective experience that arises in the soul of the individual? What is the difference between sacred and profane? What happens during sacred actions (e.g., consecration)? What is a blessing? What are Beatitudes, Sacralization and Spiritualization? What are miracles?

"This is sacred to me," means in our everyday language that something is very important and valuable to me, something I do not want to lose. In all religions, there are things, places, and people that are sacred to the faithful. Christians call the Bible "Holy Scripture" and Catholics call the Pope "Holy Father". In Catholicism, people are first beatified and then canonized according to a set ritual. However, only the Pope can canonize people among Catholics. If this happens properly in Catholicism, one can also pray to saints who may intercede with God on behalf of the faithful.

In the religious sense, the word "sacred" means to be close to God. One moves—according to the corresponding belief system—then in the sphere of the divine, the perfect or absolute. This usually involves something sublime, significant, and awe-inspiring.

The german word "heilig" (english sacred) also contains the term "heal", which means "healthy", "whole", "intact". The german word heilig probably goes back to the Old High German term "heilag", which means "favorable omen", "magic" or "luck".

In the Bible, there are also a number of (blessing) sayings that emphasize this positive side of "being whole". For example: *"May God give you what your heart desires and fulfill everything you plan"*.

12.1 The (Sometimes Hidden) Longing for the Sacred

Throughout human development, almost all cultures had some people, places, objects, or behaviors that were particularly valuable or "sacred" to the respective people. These usually included certain rituals (invocations, chants, praises, prayers, meditations, services) that were experienced and referred to as sacred.

In some form, most cultures distinguished between the *sacred* (or sacral) area and the *profane* (or worldly) area. The sacred usually belonged to another world (afterlife, spirit or god world) and was not easily and quickly accessible to everyone. Access to it was usually reserved for particularly respected people (shamans, seers, medicine men, priests) in most tribes. They were something like the connection, the channel or messenger and the contact persons into this other world of spirits and gods. With the help of these sacralized persons and certain rituals, one could ask for help from the "Otherworld" and receive messages from them. These priests were also the (gate) keepers of this spiritual world. They had a prominent role in most tribes and were often the advisors of the powerful—also in later societies. And this is still the case in many cultures today and also makes up the influence of the priests today (for more on this see: Chap. 8 Gods, Prophets, Angels, Saints, and Priests).

> **For Reflection**
> What is sacred, valuable, awe-inspiring, etc. for you? Symbolization ability: Do you have one (or more) symbols for it?

12.2 Sacredness as an Intrapsychic Phenomenon

Most people have or need something meaningful, valuable, important, or simply "sacred" in their lives. This can be tied to an idealistic, implicit life concept. Some call it "superconsciousness", "higher self" or "ideal self". Often associated with this is a feeling of awe, being moved, and the sublimity of this higher power. It may be that a whole (life) goal develops from this, which he/she (more or less consciously) strives for ("to live in the succession of Jesus Christ", "to be his apostle" etc.). This can also be a very worldly goal (more justice or solidarity) or something sacred in the spiritual-religious area, for which one is ready to make sacrifices. If this goal is highly emotionally charged, the person concerned may be ready to sacrifice his/her life in extreme cases.

The sacred is not a thing in itself, but it first arises in the mind of the person concerned.

So one can say: Sacredness is primarily an intrapsychic phenomenon. It is the inner, subjective evaluation that makes a person, place or object sacred. This arises in the heart and mind of a person—not in external reality. It is not the external circumstances, but these are only the projection surface of the internally interpreted as sacred attitude.

12.3 Group-forming Functions of Belief in Sacredness

The common belief in the sacred had (and has) a strong community-building effect for the respective group: Those who believe in it and participate in the rituals or align their lives according to it **(in-group),** belong. Those who do not believe in it are outside **(out-group).** It may be that attempts are made to convert the unbelievers to the right faith through missionary attempts. But it can also be that they are declared and fought as "enemies". This depends primarily on the "strength of belief" of each individual—i.e., how important the faith is for the individual—but also on how the "out-group" is thought and talked about in the respective religious group. But also how "the others" are dealt with. Are they—because they simply have not yet recognized and accepted the "true faith"—only seen as immature or stupid and are to be missionized? Or are they excluded as "intractable" and persecuted in the worst case?

12.4 Blessing: Support from Higher Powers

"You are a blessing for me," means in colloquial language that someone supports me, helps me and stands by my side when I am feeling bad or in need. Blessing is comfort and support, gives courage and provides backing. One can say: Blessing is the wish and help that something turns out well. This applies to the profane everyday life as well as to religious life.

There are theologians who claim that the German word "Segen" (blessing) is a derivative of the Latin word "Signum" (sign). So when we are blessed, God is supposed to give us a positive sign. Others refer more to the Latin term for blessing "benedicere": "bene" translates as good and "dicere" as say. Blessing therefore means "saying good" or "wishing good".

In the Bible, blessing is understood in such a way that the one who blesses asks his God to do something good for the recipient of the blessing, to take care of him or to protect him. In this sense, a blessing is an appeal from believers to God: Please help him, support him.

12.5 Types and Ways of Blessing

Now there are a multitude of types of blessings: from the papal grand blessing "urbi et orbi", which aims at the whole world, through the blessings in politics and society to the good wishes in private life (related to marriages, career choice, child rearing etc.). The small blessing can consist of sprinkling something with (holy) water.

There are—besides the use of holy water—a multitude of ways and manners in which blessings are given—with raised arms and open hands, hands on the head of the recipient of the blessing, sign of the cross on the forehead etc.

And there is an infinite number of blessing sayings. One of the best known is: *"The Lord bless you and keep you. He makes his face shine upon you and be gracious to you and give you peace."*

Christians say: In the blessing lies the power of God. Thus, blessing actions not only have their fixed place in services, but also in the various phases of life transition: career choice, marriage, baptism of one's own children, illnesses and dying. For believers, blessing means being accompanied by God on their journey. For this, Catholics have the seven sacraments.

12.6 Sacraments and the Grace of God

Sacraments are considered visible signs of God's grace. According to Catholicism, God himself acts through the sacraments and gives believers an earthly sign.

Sacraments are usually administered by pastors, priests, or bishops:

1. Baptism
2. Confirmation
3. Marriage
4. Eucharist/Ordination/Communion
5. Confession
6. Anointing of the Sick/Last Rites
7. Ordination (Diaconate, Priesthood, Episcopal)

The Protestant Church recognizes only two sacraments: Baptism and Communion.

12.7 Ordination

A special form of blessing is ordination. It involves blessing certain places, buildings, or objects. From the moment of ordination, these are—at least in the experience of the respective believers—particularly spiritually charged objects, which should not be "profanely misused".

12.8 The Ridiculousness of the Holy

To outsiders, what believers regard as holy often appears strange, over-the-top, incomprehensible, or even ridiculous. The transitions between holy and hypocritical are sometimes indeed fluid.

> **Heresy Objection** The counterposition to holiness is not sin, but hypocrisy. And this is not uncommon in many religious communities.

12.9 Can Everyone Bless?

The big question is: Can everyone bless? Experts disagree on this—especially the Germans, who like to have rules for everything. The great blessing is usually reserved for trained priests within the churches. In the "Framework for the Cooperation of Priests, Deacons, and Laypeople in the Field of

Liturgy," it is stated that the "small blessing" can be given by anyone who trusts that God blesses and accompanies.

Of course, the question arises: What is the difference between a great and a small blessing? Just as beauty is in the eye of the beholder, it probably depends primarily on what the recipients of the blessing think and feel.

Especially since there are now blessing-giving computer programs that spread their blessing in various devices. Just think that everyone can now call up blessings and prayers for various occasions all day long with the new Amazon Alexa Skill—including Bible verses for baptism, wedding, confirmation, and times of mourning. This skill is initiated by the Protestant Church, so it's a real "Deus ex machina" (God from the machine).

12.10 Miracles?

"Be realistic –
believe in miracles."
(Revolutionary saying)

In the current crisis times, miracles are in high demand. Not only in the religious field. The stupid thing is—you can't rely on miracles. You can wish for them, but you can't order them anywhere. They are usually unique and rarely occur in series. Of course, one could also ask: If there are miracles—why is God so sparing with miracles? And above all—why does he always show them to the wrong people?

Of course, the basic question is: Do miracles exist at all—and what do we understand by them?

Miracles are events that cause astonishment and amazement because something unexpected happens. Because the occurrence of miracles is usually inexplicable. They may be strange, magnificent and astonishing, they are simply not plausible and do not meet expectations, but perhaps even contradict the laws of nature. According to a definition by the philosopher David Hume, as early as the 18th century, one speaks of a miracle when natural laws are suspended or violated by it.

According to religious belief, the extraordinary events referred to as miracles are due to the intervention of God, who—according to the believers' view—does not have to adhere to the laws of nature.

The Bible is full of miracles. There are healing miracles, rescue miracles, food multiplication miracles, resurrection from the dead, and much more.

But reports of miracles can also be found again and again in the daily tabloid media.

About half of the population believes in miracles. Religious people do this a little more often (according to studies: Catholics 64%, Protestants even 66%). But also 43% of the non-denominational believe miracles are possible.

For children, many things that exist in the world are still miracles. The more adult they become, the less they are impressed by what they once called miracles. A wise person said: Miracles only exist for people who (still) do not understand.

It is certain: It would be a miracle if there were miracles.

> **For Reflection**
> Can you still truly marvel?
>   Try to simply perceive something without immediately putting it into words. Then you might already experience a small miracle …

12.11 Enjoying the Moment

With or without blessing or miracle, it is certainly a skill to enjoy the moment—and to bless it, if you like. But—if you break it down a bit and leave out all the spiritual brimborium, you can say, all sincerely meant good wishes are a blessing. With or without God.

"God grant me the serenity,
to accept the things I cannot change,
the courage,
to change the things I can,
and the wisdom,
to distinguish one from the other."

References

Buggle, Franz: Denn sie wissen nicht, was sie glauben, Aschaffenburg 2004 (alibri)
James, William: Die Vielfalt religiöser Erfahrung, Olten 1979 (Walter)
Kolbe, Christoph: Heilung oder Hindernis—Religion bei Freud, Adler, Fromm, Jung und Frankl, Stuttgart 1986 (Kreuz)

Linnewedel, Jürgen: Mystik—Meditation—Yoga—Zen, Stuttgart 1975 (Quell)

Mursell, Gordon: Die Geschichte der Christlichen Spiritualität, Stuttgart 2002 (Kreuz)

Schmelzer, Carsten St.: Heilung—Was wir glauben und erwarten dürfen, Witten 2013 (SCM-Brockhaus)

Zohar, D. Marshall, I.: SQ—Spirituelle Intelligenz, Bern/München/Wien 1999, (Scherz)

Part IV

The Light and Dark Sides of Religion

13

Humanistic and Authoritarian Religion: Salvation and Disaster Through Faith

Summary

This chapter deals with the light- and shadow sides of religions. The psychoanalyst Erich Fromm distinguished very early between authoritarian and humanistic religion. It is about the question, where is religion supportive and helpful for the development of humans—and where is it harmful, because it disempowers and hinders the free development of humans. It also deals with the question of what religion is used for and how power is exercised with religion.

13.1 The Difference Between Authoritarian and Humanistic Religion

The distinction between authoritarian and humanistic religion runs—according to Erich Fromm's view—through all religions. All creeds can have authoritarian or even totalitarian traits or develop in that direction. This applies to extreme forms such as fanatical Islamism (see the current terrorist attacks by Islamist attackers). But there are also these excesses in Christianity: e.g., the armed conflicts between Catholic and Protestant Christians in Northern Ireland.

The distinction between authoritarian and humanistic religion can also be found in the milder forms of religious conflicts. Because the transitions between faith certainty, dogmatism, proselytizing, fanaticism and terrorism are fluid.

13.2 Authoritarian Religion: From Good News and Threats

Authoritarian Religion is (according to Erich Fromm) characterized by the idea that a higher power (God) has a claim to worship, adoration, and obedience. The essential point is the submission of humans to the (supposed) power of God. This power can be transferred to a human leader (as a representative of God on earth), i.e., to leaders of religious communities or "true" interpreters of the Holy Books (Bible, Quran, Talmud …): Priests, gurus, mullahs, bishops, the pope thus receive unquestionable power. It is not allowed to question this and to distance oneself from the belief system. The following criteria characterize authoritarian religions:

- Dualistic view of God and the world (Good/Evil, Black/White)
- The deity is omniscient and omnipotent
- Humans are fundamentally powerless and insignificant
- They gain their strength only through submission to the unquestionable religious dogmas and the dogmatic ideas of the religious community
- Only willing submission to the power of God leads to his grace/help
- The main virtue is obedience
- The main sin is disobedience
- Predominant mood: Fear, guilt, suffering, anxiety
- Loss of independence and integrity as an individual
- They surrender the responsibility for their life to God
- Psychological gain: Awe-inspiring power protects me, I am part of it (the good) and have my role in "God's work"

13.3 Humanistic Religion

According to Erich Fromm, humanistic religion is characterized by the feeling of oneness with the universe. Self-realization (and not submission) is what humans aim to achieve in humanistic religion. Fromm writes: "Faith is the certainty of conviction, acquired through one's own experience by means of thinking and feeling, not acceptance of a doctrine on the basis of the prestige of the one who established it." For him, the predominant mood is joy. Humanistic religion does not prescribe how we should live. Humans have the freedom—without religious guidelines—to find out who they are, what is inherent in them, and what wants to be realized in them. This also gives them responsibility for their lives. Humanistic religion is characterized by the following points:

- The focus is on the human who affirms his powers and strengths.
- He develops reason to understand himself and his fellow human beings.
- Self-realization (not obedience) is a virtue.
- Self-knowledge and self-experience aim to know one's own possibilities and limits.
- And to take responsibility for one's own actions.
- To develop love for others, oneself, and the "universe".
- Good faith is the sure conviction through tested experience in thinking and feeling, not by adopting doctrines or belief in authorities.
- Independence and free decision are allowed (as well as making mistakes).
- Predominant is an integrated view of God and the world.

The common denominator is found in Immanuel Kant's statement: *"Have the courage to use your own understanding."*

Religions become problematic and dangerous when they become dogmatic and rigid and no longer perceive reality and try to distort reality on the Procrustean bed of their belief system. Sometimes it is therefore helpful to take a closer look at and clear out the burden of religious dogmas that have accumulated over the history of religion. Good religion is not worship of the ashes, but carrying forward the fire. In Islam it is said: "Trust in Allah, but tie your camel."

References

Bucher, Anton A.: Psychologie der Spiritualität, Weinheim 2007 (Beltz)
Fromm, Erich: Haben oder Sein, München 1976 (dtv)
Fromm, Erich, Suzuki, de Martino: Zen-Buddhismus und Psychoanalyse, Frankfurt 1972 (Suhrkamp)
Utsch, M., Bonelli, R. M., Pfeifer, S.: Psychotherapie und Spiritualität, Berlin/Heidelberg 2014 (Springer)

14

How Religion and Faith Become a Problematic Cult: Criteria for Sects

> **Summary**
>
> This chapter deals with the problematic aspects of religion, as they are primarily practiced in religious special organizations (sects, psycho groups, esoteric scene etc.). How do people get into these religious communities? What attracts them? Who is at risk of falling into these groups? How are the members bound? What is the internal structure of these groups? What techniques of personality change are used to influence the individual group member?

In addition to the traditional major churches, there are said to be around 300 religious special communities, "sects" and problematic cults in Germany with 1.5–2.5 million members—and new ones are constantly being formed. More and more "mini-gurus" and "eso-coaches" feel called to earn their money with their consulting offers on the psycho market and in the esoteric scene. In uncertain times, "illusion sellers" are booming. More or less absurd ideas are propagated in the scene, more or less absurd methods and techniques are practiced there. And a lot of money is made with it. "Sects", destructive cults and the esoteric scene—as reported by the media—are experiencing an unbroken influx. So what, one might say, the world is big enough for everyone to be wrong in their own way. If only it were that simple …

14.1 Who Ends Up in Which Religious Community, Becomes at Home or Bound There?

How a person ends up in a problematic group (this can be a "sect" or even a marginal group within the major churches) is always a highly individual process. Some are looking for a system of meaning, others are disappointed with traditional religions and/or disoriented. Often it happens in personal crisis situations, in which the people concerned no longer know what to do and are looking for ways out and/or the previous support systems have failed for them. The following groups of people can be distinguished in this context.

14.2 Seekers

These are people who are looking for a different life. They may hope for a new meaning in their life, want more intense self-experience, "consciousness expansion", adventure, border experiences. Often there is a desire for self-discovery, for a drastic change in life ("transformation") or even a "rebirth of the true human".

14.3 Disappointed

Here you will find people with a high protest potential, who are dissatisfied with their life, society or even the world as a whole. Here the feeling often prevails: "I am living the wrong life."

14.4 Disoriented

These are people who cannot cope with the complexity of life in our time. They desire simple, clear rules to guide their lives.

14.5 People in Acute Personal Crises

These can be extreme puberty crises, the currently hotly debated "quarter-life crisis", the much invoked "midlife crisis", or sudden unemployment, divorce, death of a relative etc. can be triggers.

14.6 People with Severe Mental Problems

Particularly at risk are people who have had bad experiences with the traditional support system (psychiatry, three-minute medicine …) and who cling to any straw that somehow promises hope.

14.7 Fit

Surely these subgroups are not cleanly separable from each other. There are transitions and commonalities between these groups of people. Since the process is highly individual, it is worth looking very closely at each individual person. So one can ask:

> Which **person**
> - with what genetic-constitutional equipment,
> - with what life history,
> - grew up in which family (with what religious traditions),
> - with what unresolved conflicts, injuries, and blockages,
> - with what undeveloped sides and deficits,
> - with what experiences (in school, puberty, profession, adulthood),
> - with what lifestyle and philosophy …,

> is addressed by which **sect/church/group/religion**
> - with what kind of offer,
> - with what advertising strategies,

in what current **situation**

- and mental,
- physical,
- social condition

Here the highly individual situation in which each individual person has fallen into one of the groups is revealed. This is called the **fit.** This can happen to one person in a very short time ("snapping") and for another person it can be a lengthy process ("shaping") that can take months.

> **Heresy Objection** Some people who seek God do not find him, but find some comic joke figure off the shelf, which are offered by the various religious communities on the market of worldviews—whether they are called Krishna, Jehovah, Allah or Jesus Christ. And once you're hooked, it's not easy to get rid of the gentlemen. It's about as difficult as trying to get rid of a protracted, chronic syphilis. The figures stick to one like superglue—if you're not careful, for all eternity.

14.8 Criteria for Assessing Spiritual Groups in the Esoteric Scene and Psycho Market

In this it is certainly not every spiritual or alternative group that is problematic per se. And certainly not all sects are the same, psycho cults are the same. The esoteric and sect scene is a confusing jungle that is constantly changing and producing new blooms.

Often, however, the criteria for assessing such groups are lacking: What exactly makes a group problematic or even dangerous?

What makes it a "destructive cult" that makes people dependent, exploits or destroys them? What are the mechanisms by which this happens?

On the other hand, how can it be recognized whether a "sect hunt" is not interest-driven panic-mongering by traditional institutions (such as the churches) who are losing members?

Precisely because the field is so confusing and the groups are so different from each other, it is necessary to find objective criteria for a differentiated assessment, almost a grid, in order to create a "profile" of the respective group (in relation to its problematic or dangerous nature). The following checklist is intended to serve this purpose. It is divided into six areas that can become problem areas (or have already become) in the individual groups:

1. Ideology
2. The central figure
3. Group structure
4. Influence on the member
5. Techniques of personality change
6. Contacts to the outside and dealing with former members and critics

14.8.1　Ideology: Theory, Belief, Goals

Here it is about the theoretical background of the group. Because not only the practice, but also the ideological orientation can lead to various problems—especially when the following tendencies prevail:

- **"Overvalued Idea":** Paradise on earth or the "new human" can be created in the short term using the doctrine (delusions of grandeur, megalomania).
- **Monopoly of Truth:** The group has (in their opinion) the only valid world explanation system.
- **Black-and-White Thinking:** Simple good-evil or right-wrong patterns shape thinking and action.
- **End Time Vision:** The end of the world is near (for non-believers).
- **Rescue Plan:** There are patent recipes in the group that promise salvation (only for believers).
- **Expansive Claim to Power:** "We must save the world" is the tenor.

14.8.2　The Central Figure: Leader, Master, Saint, Guru

Here, the following points should be noted:

- **Cult of the Leader:** He/she is revered as God, Saint, or "Channel" (who has a direct line to God or is God's representative on earth). He/she is omnipotent, clairvoyant, or has miraculous abilities.
- **Leadership Style:** He/she has supreme (no longer criticizable) authority, demands uncritical loyalty, and claims the monopoly of truth.
- **Charismatization:** Veneration of saints and the propagation of idealizing legends are promoted.

14.8.3 Group Structure: Elite Community

Here, the following points are in the foreground:

- **Isolation from the Outside:** The group is a closed system with rigid external boundaries.
- **High Group Cohesion:** The group sticks together "like tar and sulfur", monitors, controls, and punishes each other. There may be an internal special language.
- There exists a **steep hierarchy** with command authority of the superiors, obedience of the simple member, and a tiered information system.
- **Elite Consciousness:** Group members feel like the avant-garde to save the world/humanity. The compulsion to proselytize and/or martyr ideology shape the group consciousness.
- **Exploitation:** Group members allow themselves to be exploited (more or less voluntarily) materially or/and as cheap labor.
- **Subversive and Illegal Activities:** The group believes it is above the law and pushes members (openly or covertly) to illegal activities (blackmailability!).

14.8.4 Influence on the Member: Mind Control

This area deals with the personal, individual levels of influence:

- **Deindividualization:** Total devotion is demanded, the group and the common goal are more important than the individual.
- **Influence on everyday life is high:** There are regulations for eating, clothing, personal hygiene, daily routine, exit and contact bans, telephone and mail controls. Relationships and sexuality are regulated.
- **Material Dependence:** The group member has no private property and/or no money. They are not (or very poorly) paid for their work and they are not insured for sickness, accident or pension. Passport, driver's license, etc. are kept together.
- **Magical Thinking** prevails in the group: "Everything is predestined", "God wants it that way".
- **Break with personal life history:** Relationships with the family of origin, partners and friends are broken off. School, studies, profession are given up. The previous life history is reinterpreted.

- **Cult Identity:** The group member gets a new name, moves almost exclusively in the group and undergoes a gradual "revaluation of all values" . This is accompanied by a loss of reality and suitability for a life outside the group. Massive psychological dependence develops.

14.8.5 Techniques for Personality Change

- **Emotion-mobilizing, euphoric and consciousness-altering techniques** are used: Hyperventilation, chanting, drugs, speaking in tongues, excessive meditation etc.
- **Repeated destabilization** through fasting, sleep deprivation, physical and psychological overexertion, sensory deprivation etc.
- The goal is a kind of **"spiritual experience",** which is then interpreted by the group as the birth of the true human being ("Finally, I have found myself.").

14.8.6 External Contacts and Dealing with Former Members and Critics

- The group practices **manipulative recruitment methods**, in which people are lured with unrealistic promises.
- **Bunker Mentality:** The group massively isolates itself ("Inside heaven, outside hell"). Conspiracy theories and paranoia prevail.
- There is **no legitimate reason to leave the group;** therefore, former members are declared non-persons ("outlawed", contact break), who are sometimes blackmailed.
- **Critics are intimidated** and attempts are made to silence them with threats, public defamation, telephone terror, lawsuits or even physical attacks.

The present checklist allows a differentiated assessment of religious groups in the esoteric and psycho-market and sect scene according to a number of objective criteria. Individual characteristics listed do not necessarily make a group conflict-prone or dangerous, as they can also be found in other associations.

Groups are more problematic the more critical points apply to them. If a profile emerges from many existing individual characteristics, one can speak of a destructive cult.

References

Bohnke, Ben-Alexander: Esoterik—Die Welt des Geheimen, Düsseldorf 1991 (Econ)
Caberta, Ursula: Schwarzbuch Esoterik, Gütersloh 2010 (Gütersloher Verlagshaus)
Deutscher Bundestag: Abschlussbericht der Enquete-Kommission "Sogenannte Sekten und Psychogruppen", Bonn 1998 (Ref. Öffentlichkeitsarbeit)
Gross, Werner (Eds.): Psychomarkt, Sekten, Destruktive Kulte (2. ed), Bonn 1996 (Deutscher Psychologen Verlag)
Goldner, Colin: Psycho—Therapien zwischen Seriosität und Scharlatanerie, Augsburg 1997 (Pattloch)
Gross, Werner: Sucht ohne Drogen, Frankfurt 2003 (Fischer-TB)
Hutten, Kurt: Seher, Grübler, Enthusiasten, Stuttgart 1982 (Quell)
Kramer, J., Alstad, D.: Die Guru Papers—Masken der Macht, Frankfurt 1995 (Verlag 2001)
Nordhausen, F., Billerbeck, L. v.: Psycho-Sekten—Die Praktiken der Seelenfänger, Berlin 1997 (Ch. Links)
Poppelreuter, St., Gross, W. (Eds.): Nicht nur Drogen machen süchtig, Weinheim 2000 (Psychologie Verlags Union)
Pohl, Sarah: Spiritueller Schiffbruch? Sich selbst und anderen in Sinnnot helfen, Göttingen 2022 (Vandenhoeck & Ruprecht)
Schorsch, Christof: Die New Age-Bewegung, Gütersloh 1988 (Gütersloher Verlagshaus)
Schneider, Wolf: Kleines Lexikon esoterischer Irrtümer, Gütersloh 2008 (Gütersloher Verlagshaus)
Singer, Margaret, Taler: Sekten—Wie Menschen Ihre Freiheit verlieren und wiedergewinnen können, Heidelberg 1997 (Carl Auer)
Schwertfeger, Bärbel: Der Griff nach der Psyche, Frankfurt 1998 (Campus)
Scheurlen, Paul: Die Sekten der Gegenwart, Stuttgart 1930 (Quell)
Stamm, Hugo: Sekten—Im Bann von Sucht und Macht, Zürich 1995 (Kreuz)

15

Health-promoting and Disease-causing Religiosity

> **Summary**
> This chapter deals with healthy and harmful religiosity. Where is religiosity beneficial for the individual, and where is it harmful because it hinders the free and healthy development of the individual.

"The blind man is a good guide in the dark night."
"During the day, one should rely on one's own eyes."

How do we want and how should we live? As it concerns the fundamental questions of being human, a religious worldview not only influences the individual construction of reality (Who am I? What am I doing here? What is a meaningful life for me?), but also well-being. Because undoubtedly, religion and faith can have an impact on a person's state of mind and health. This can be positive, but also problematic. And this depends both on the content of faith and the strength of faith.

If God is experienced as a benevolent, supportive, and loving force, this has positive effects—especially in times of fate and crisis, many find "trust in God" helpful. However, if a punishing and judging image of God prevails, this has negative results.

So one can say that the current subjective attitude and processing of the religion learned and practiced in one's life history are important in the specific situation.

So one cannot say: Catholicism is good and Protestantism is bad or Islam is good and Buddhism is bad, but it depends on what one makes of one's faith on the subjective "inner stage". And this depends both on the content of faith and the intensity of faith. And last but not least, it is about the question of what role religion plays in my life in general and how far it has played a role in the construction and development of my personality structure.

A meta-study, in which about 850 study results on the topic "Does religion make you healthy or sick?" were summarized in an overview (Koenig et al. 2001, according to Marion Schowalter, Würzburg), came to the following result:

15.1 Religion Makes You Healthy …

- When religion is seen as a real **resource**
- Serious believers suffer less from depression, anxiety, and addiction
- They have a **lower risk of illness**
- They **recover better** after illnesses
- Religion carries believers in times of need, provides **hope and orientation**
- Gives the feeling of being **supported** in difficult life situations. They usually live by the life motto "You are not alone"
- In general, believers have a **better way of dealing with suffering,** they have a higher well-being, their self-healing powers are higher, and they have better stress management
- They have a **higher life satisfaction**
- They are **more empathetic, attentive, and compassionate**
- They have **less fear of death**

Important: Only religious patients benefit from religious interventions!!!

15.2 Religion Makes You Sick …

- Religion can **distort internally**
- Religion can make people **dependent,** conform them and produce fear in them
- Often one finds **lack of joy in life** in religious people ("Duty is more important than fun")
- Religious people often direct **their anger against themselves**
- Religion can produce **illusions instead of hope**

- **Miracles** are not everyday occurrences and cannot be produced by religious rituals (prayers, vows, services …)
- High "ego—ideal: A **"terror of the religious ego ideal"** can arise ("following Jesus")
- High **social pressure and exclusion:** Fear of punishment
- **Cognitive rigidity:** rigid, inflexible
- **Strict moral guidelines:** Ecclesiogenic neuroses
- **Belief in the omnipotence of God:** Passivity towards God
- **Theory of divine action:** Permanent threat
- **Negative emotions:** Fear, depression, addiction
- **Idealization of alternative values:** "Everything is better than the church"

15.3 Perishing from Faith: Mental Illnesses Caused by Religion

- The risk of mental illness is particularly high if the person has an image of God that is punishing and controlling: God of revenge, God of judgement, God of accounting, God of performance, etc.
- When the threat (or fear) of disaster predominates and is more significant than the message of salvation
- When there is a risk of losing realistic assessments, boundaries, and proportions
- When religion leads to isolation and individualization and the person in question is (unfiltered) exposed to his inner processes and there is no corrective from the outside. Then the following can occur:
- Obsessive-compulsive disorders
- Depressions
- Fears
- Religious neuroses
- Physical illnesses/Psychosomatic disorders
- Personality disorders
- Addiction
- Psychoses/Delusions

References

Booth, Leo: Wenn Gott zur Droge wird, München 1999 (Kösel)

Bragdon, Emma: Spirituelle Krisen—Wendepunkte im Leben, Freiburg 1991 (Bauer)

Hark, Helmut: Religiöse Neurosen, Stuttgart 1984 (Kreuz)

Harris, Marvin: Fauler Zauber—unsere Sehnsucht nach der anderen Welt, Stuttgart 1993 (Klett-Cotta)

Linke, Detlef B.: Religion als Risiko—Geist, Glaube und Gehirn, Reinbek 2005 (Rowohlt)

Moser, Tilmann: Gottesvergiftung, Frankfurt 1976 (Suhrkamp)

Scharfetter, Christian: Der spirituelle Weg und seine Gefahren, Stuttgart 1999 (Thieme)

Tempelmann, Inge: Geistlicher Missbrauch—Auswege aus frommer Gewalt, Wuppertal 2007 (Brockhaus)

Part V

Conclusion: Globalization - From Deluge to Flood of Meaning

16

Trust and Faith—What Really Helps (And What Harms)

> **Summary**
>
> This chapter deals with the fundamental questions of human life and philosophy: What purpose do we have in our life? How do we find it? What role do religions play in this? Where do they help? When do they become problematic and restrictive?

16.1 The Meaning of Crises

Some questions we do not seek—they come to us unasked: in times of crisis, when we are stuck in a dead end, when problems overwhelm us (diseases, pain, separations, death …). Often we only then ask about the meaning. Why is this happening to us? Why me? Why now?

As if we were torn from our somnambulistic security in which we have so far walked, tumbled or swam through life, and suddenly wake up to think about the meaning. What does a fish know about the water in which it swims? It might be similar with us humans: What does man know about his purpose in life? Because in our society, the crises of meaning, the rampant loss of meaning, and the inner unfulfillment are omnipresent.

Perhaps crises serve this purpose: In crises, we sometimes have to ask very fundamental questions about what we have so far taken for granted. It's like waking up from a dream: What am I actually doing in my everyday routine? How do I spend my lifetime? Do I actually want this? Is it good? Does it do me good? Am I doing something good? Meaning-making is a process. It is sometimes laborious, but fulfilling. And meaning makes us resilient.

"He who has a why to live,
can bear almost any how."
(Viktor Frankl, Viennese psychiatrist,
who survived a concentration camp)

Meaning is more than just pleasure and quick satisfaction. Meaning extends beyond us. It also involves other people or beings, perhaps even the world. If I leave the world a little better than I found it—even if it's only by 0.1 mm—then that can make sense. If I do something good for others, if I do something for nature, then that can make sense. One could call it generativity (creating something of lasting value). A good life for me is a **sensual life** and a **meaningful life.** It requires external success and inner fulfillment—in each case in very different and individual expression and mixture.

The question of meaning is probably as old as humanity. Since the time when our brain development was so advanced that we could develop something like consciousness, we have asked ourselves what all this actually means, why we are here, what we are supposed to do here, what our task is—and how free we can decide how we live.

So, the big questions of humanity are found here. And religions effortlessly and quickly provide answers—without us having to think about it ourselves. Thus, we adopt—because we have learned it this way and everyone in our environment does it this way—religious systems of meaning off the shelf out of laziness and convenience. It is important: Do not swallow the fish with the bones and do not accept what sticks in your throat. Measure the beliefs against reality. It is not a betrayal of faith to give it up—because you know better.

It may be that life has no meaning—but it is also certain that we can give life a meaning. And perhaps that is even our duty if we cannot or do not want to adopt a religious system of meaning. In the interest of life—which system of world explanation would be helpful for this?

16.2 No Power to Dogmas: Wisdom Instead of Belief

"Insanity is
the inability to doubt."
(Peter Ustinov)

Thus, one can also describe religions as bridges into the intrapsychic void. If one is able to walk them with hope, they can be healing—but also dangerous. The transitions between hope and illusion are fluid. Undoubtedly, religions can be helpful for believers—even if they are illusions. Because it is about the subjective feeling of basic trust and not about religious dogmas.

Basic Trust Instead of Belief
The goal could thus be exactly this basic trust. One could also say finding home in infinity—and that, without being naive. However, the thing with transcendence is also not entirely harmless—especially if one thinks that with a few externally performed rituals (prayers, mantras, church visits, physical exercises) one has already made it and found a lasting escape from the daily grind and the daily setbacks. The question is whether this escape will still work tomorrow. In the mystical traditions it is said: "Stand firm in this world and only then lean towards the other."

16.3 Spiritual Wanderers

> *"Respect people,*
> *who seek truth and meaning.*
> *Be careful with those,*
> *who claim to have found them."*

Probably, we humans are wanderers in search—driven by the primal longing for security and meaning. In this process, many people believe all sorts of things. The important aid is probably **not so much what** they believe, but the way **how** they believe and what their belief gives them. After all, we humans are "meaning-needy beings of deficiency". While we used to unquestioningly adopt the faith lived in our birth region (absorbed quasi with mother's milk), today it is much more complicated. Because we live in a multi-option society, in which a multitude of religions and sense systems worldwide compete with each other and rush upon us as a real "flood of meaning". The unique true and universally valid belief has long been lost to us. Perhaps that is why many have now become "spiritual wanderers"—in search of the meaning of life that suits us. And this meaning of life is not easy to find, because it requires a certain degree of self-reflection and we may have to go through various stages (full of errors and confusions) on the way there, without knowing whether we will ever finally arrive. After all, the world is big enough for everyone (in his own way) to be wrong on it.

Nowadays (at least in our regions) everyone has a choice: One is not at the mercy of the religion one grew up with. It does not have to accompany us (or even dominate us) for a lifetime. Here too, Kant's sentence applies: "Dare to use your own understanding"—and to choose which worldview is right for you and suits you.

However, one does not have to have a clearly defined belief to lead a good life: Because—whether it suits the believers or not:

"The gates of paradise are always open to unbelievers."

16.4 Reason Against Dogmas

"Science without religion is lame,
religion without science is blind."
(Albert Einstein)

Against the true core of religions—namely developing basic trust, giving hope, without making illusions—there is nothing to say. The problems begin with the dogmas of the faith of the individual religious systems, namely when one clings to one's own truth and considers it the only right and true one and devalues or even fights all others.

Even if the contents of faith are seen by many as madness, nonsense and rubbish, the effects that religions produce in individual believers are strikingly positive: With the help of religions, some get away from alcohol or heroin, give themselves a sense of life again from the darkest depressions or even hold back from suicide through prayers.

16.5 Hope Instead of Illusion

A blind man is a good guide in the night. When it is bright, one should rather use their own eyes. Some prefer not to open their eyes and rather be guided. Others want no one else to open their eyes—then they can guide better. They also do not want those being guided to use their brains. Do not let them stop you: If you have a brain—use it.

"Hope is not optimism.
It is not the conviction that something will turn out well,
but the certainty that something makes sense
– regardless of how it turns out."
(Václav Havel)

I have so much hope: In the long run, reason will always triumph over illusions, dogmas, and tradition.

References

Brantschen, Niklaus: Gottlos beten, Ostfildern 2022 (Patmos-Verlag)
Bucher, Anton A.: Psychologie der Spiritualität, Weinheim 2007 (Beltz)
Frankl, Viktor E.: Der Wille zum Sinn – Bern 1972, 2. Auflage (Huber)
Hellinger, Bert: Religion, Psychotherapie, Seelsorge, München 2000 (Kösel)
Moser, Tilmann: Gott auf der Couch, Gütersloh 2011 (Gütersloher Verlagshaus)
Sölle, Dorothee: Den Rhythmus des Lebens spüren, Freiburg 2001 (Herder Spektrum)
Sölle, Dorothee: Atheistisch an Gott glauben, Olten/CH 1968 (Walter)
Utsch, M., Bonelli, R. M., Pfeifer, S.: Psychotherapie und Spiritualität, Berlin/Heidelberg 2014 (Springer)
Wiesenhütter, Eckart: Religion und Tiefenpsychologie, Gütersloh 1977 (Gütersloher Verlagshaus)
Zohar, D. Marshall, I.: SQ – Spirituelle Intelligenz, Bern/München/Wien 1999 (Scherz)

17

Theses: Sense and Nonsense of Religion and Religiosity

17.1 World Explanation Systems

- Religions are world explanation and meaning systems
- They are symbolizations of primal trust and useful providers of hope—but sometimes also harmful illusion producers
- Religions usually consider themselves the only true, eternal, and final world explanation and meaning system

17.2 Levels of Interpretation

- Religions are interpretations of neurological states, psychological experiences, and social attributions. They are attempts to express the inexpressible, to make the incomprehensible comprehensible *(e.g., death)*
- Religiosity structures, concretizes, and manifests diffuse-subjective inner truths and experiences of reality and provides interpretations by linking these experiences with external images of God *(Christ, Krishna, Allah, Jehovah, etc.)* and assuming that the external image saves people
- Religions are attempts to codify primal trust in words, symbols, and ritual instructions. They can be signposts, but they are not the goal and result

17.3 Origin of Religions

- The origin of all religions is fear, emptiness, meaninglessness, death, the unboundness of humans *(Contrast: instinctual certainty of animals)*
- **Background:** Humans are unfinished "physiological preterm births"—only through this do we have a space for questions of meaning. This space was (initially) replaced by religious world explanations. It is easier to adopt a ready-made system of meaning than to think about it oneself.

17.4 God is a Human Idea

- All religions and religious rules are made by humans. The more they correspond to nature, the more "human" (and natural) they are and the longer they will endure
- Because God/gods only live in the brains of their believers and because they are made by humans, God is ultimately a human idea
- With an image of God, people create through dogmas an unquestionable authority that provides support, (supposedly) clear orientation, and security. This is important both intrapsychically and socio-psychologically and socially

17.5 Primal Trust vs. Faith

- Primal trust instead of faith: Faith—in the sense of primal trust—is sensible, health-promoting, and useful
- Faith has a content that one can (must) believe. Primal trust does not need dogmas, prescriptions, and rules
- Faith is subjective truth (or inter-subjective—among the group of believers), but never objective truth

17.6 Certainty and Dogmatism

- The smaller (or more confused) the mind, the more concrete must be the image of God, religion, and (faith-)certainty

- Those who take symbols (relics) + religious actions (blessings, pilgrimages) too seriously, run the risk of kitsch, magical thinking, and delusional systems: Every concrete religion is more or less a "pseudo-religion"
- Fundamentalism is a manifestation of missionary-aggressive religious practice with a claim to absoluteness
- Dogmatism is stupidity coupled with fear, aggression, and possibly fanaticism: Possessed or inspired?
- Spiritual experiences are experiences of boundary dissolution and often resemble psychosis (causes of faith certainty?)

17.7 Subjectively and Objectively True

- Belief is a highly subjective event: Just as beauty is in the eye of the beholder, the sacred arises in the head/heart of the person—not in external reality.
- What happens on the "inner stage" is central. What happens on the "outer stage" of different belief systems is interchangeable.

17.8 What, How, and Why

- It's not so much about **what** you believe, but about **how** you believe (and **why**)
- The healing aspect of faith has little to do with the image of God *(Jesus, Krishna, Allah)*, faith content *(Bible, Quran, Vedas, Talmud)* or faith system *(Christianity, Hinduism, Islam, Buddhism, Judaism)* (i.e., **what** I believe), but with the degree of mobilization of basic trust (i.e., **how** I believe)
- You don't need a religion to be a good person and moral

17.9 Knowledge and Belief

- Knowledge makes free and secure, belief makes dependent ("Do you already know or do you still believe … "—Giordano Bruno Foundation)
- Unfortunately, you can't know everything. Science alone cannot explain the world—and it does not warm
- However: **Unreflected** belief is the philosophy of the stupid and lazy

17.10 Paradigm Shift: Time and Globalization

- Religions are world explanation systems that provide an answer to questions of meaning for a specific, limited time, which—although always with a claim to eternity—may be right for today and not tomorrow …
- Due to globalization, the various religions have lost their monopoly position as the only valid world explanation system: Where they differ, the "culturally or zeitgeist-shaped (non-)sense" begins
- Therefore, it makes sense to distinguish between ethical-moral values (which are more or less the same in all world religions) and pure faith content
- **"Benchmarking"**: The religions of the 3rd millennium will ideally be universal, globally transcultural, undogmatic, boundless (with local/individual expressions)—or the religions will (through missionizing, fanaticizing) clash in the "Clash of the cultures" …

17.11 Use and Abuse

- Religions and beliefs were (and still are) used and abused to keep people dependent and small, to terrorize and even kill them. They had a kind of monopoly on the exploitation of idealism for centuries—especially of young people.
- Churches today are only rudimentary faith communities. Many sects and churches are religiously neglected and run down.
- Today, they are often perceived by many people as institutions preventing real basic trust.
- Today, they are primarily power institutions and instruments of power, which are instrumentalized by certain societal forces and interest groups. Their original task is often only secondary: Almost all religions have at some point become whores of the powerful (Prince to Bishop: "You keep them stupid, I keep them poor.").

17.12 Gods and Wars

- When the gods clash, people die en masse: Many wars have arisen because of dogmatic certainties of faith and the contents of faith. As long as God has to serve as the cause of murder, manslaughter, war and people are killed in his name, the old religions remain unbelievable

17.13 Misuse and Demolition Houses

- Because religious organizations have misused faith for so long *("Opium for the people")*, they are for many only demolition houses, from which one can break out one or the other useful thing *("Patchwork religiosity")*
- Overall, most religions, churches, and faith communities are based on outdated (faith) foundations

17.14 Futility and Tolerance

- It is not to be excluded, that (human) life has no meaning. What is certain is that we can give it a meaning. This does not have to be a transcendent or religious system of meaning "off the peg".
- Today we have choices—therefore:
- Tolerance: The world is big enough for everyone to be wrong in their own way
- After all: What can we really know?

17.15 Distance to One's Own Worldview

- The goal is to develop basic trust and learn to stand firmly in the air with both feet
- The development should go towards the inner core of all religions, the mystical dimension
- It is certainly helpful to develop distance to one's own worldview and critical reflection.

References

Bucher, Anton A.: Psychologie der Spiritualität, Weinheim 2007 (Beltz)

Brantschen, Niklaus: Gottlos beten, Ostfildern 2022 (Patmos-Verlag)

Frankl, Viktor E.: Die Sinnfrage in der Psychotherapie, München 1981 (Piper)

Jarzombek, Dieter (Hrsg.): Freiheit, die wir meinen, Berlin 2014 (Lit-Verlag Dr. W. Hopf)

Metz, Wulf (Hrsg): Handbuch Weltreligionen, Wuppertal 2003, 5. Aufl. (Brockhaus)

Nozick, Robert: Vom richtigen, guten und glücklichen Leben, München 1993 (DTV)

Rensch, Bernhard: Das universelle Weltbild, Frankfurt 1977 (Fischer-TB)

Smith, Huston: Eine Wahrheit, viele Wege – Die großen Religionen der Welt, Freiburg 1993 (Bauer)

Sölle, Dorothee: Atheistisch an Gott glauben, Olten/CH 1968 (Walter)

Utsch, M., Bonelli, R. M., Pfeifer, S.: Psychotherapie und Spiritualität, Berlin/Heidelberg 2014 (Springer)

18

Epilogue: With Both Feet Firmly in the Air

> **Summary**
>
> This chapter is the conclusion and the final thoughts of the book. It addresses the fundamental questions: What meaning do I give to my life? What is the purpose of religions? Where do they help? When do they become problematic and restrictive? What is the difference between knowledge and belief? What will remain of religions? What does the future of religions look like? What systems of meaning will we develop in the future?

*"Even if one does not believe in God,
one should live as if one did."*
(Max Perutz, Nobel laureate for Biochemistry)

The curtain is closed—and all questions are open? No, not quite: Because religiosity has to do with the innermost core of a person, which is to a considerable extent unconscious. Religions are hypotheses. Some of them are unverifiable, many are falsified, few are verified. As long as religion remains vague, diffuse, and thus open to many interpretations, it is successful. When it becomes concrete, it often starts to falter.

And what does each individual do with it? Even if a residual doubt remains—how should one deal with the question of meaning? Ultimately: How well does one live without illusions?

After all, the background of religiosity is largely subjective (and collective) unconscious: What does a fish know about the water in which it swims? What does a person know about the faith by which he lives? The only way to this is self-reflection and conscious confrontation with it. Look closely and don't swallow the fish with all its bones.

Are we really heroic masters and determiners of our fate or are we just fulfilling a divine plan intended for us? Or are we just the "fleas on the back of the Leviathan" and victims of unpredictable evolution? What can a person really recognize and know about himself and his purpose? And because this is so largely unconscious, it also partly explains the radicalism with which the certainty of faith of the religious is sometimes represented: Especially when I am unsure in my deepest heart, I have to convince myself that I am very sure, by acting outwardly as if I were an impregnable fortress of faith. Therefore, I must not allow other beliefs that question my only true view. Thus, fear becomes dogmatism and perhaps even fanaticism, which in the worst case ends in religious wars. It is clear: One can sacrifice one's life for an idea, a belief - but only one's own, not that of (many) others.

Are traditional religions part of the problem or part of the solution? Probably both, depending on how they are used.

> **Heretical Objection** One can and may invent all sorts of fantasies. One can also develop all sorts of matching theories. However, they should be able to withstand the reality test. That is, they must not contradict the proven findings of the sciences.

"Religion can help, religion can harm." This quote begins an article in the "Journal for Religion and Worldview" (4/2023, p. 284), published by the Protestant Central Office for Worldview Questions. And the article continues: "After the health-promoting effects of positive beliefs and practices have been proven in the German-speaking world, reports are increasing about the effects of toxic communities, religious violence or spiritual abuse." Here the two sides of religion are shown: The brighter the light, the darker the shadow. Or: The holier the festival, the busier the devil.

A blind man is a good guide in the night. When it is light, one should rather use one's eyes. However: Some people do not want to open their eyes and prefer to be led. Others want no one but themselves to open their eyes—then they can lead better. They also do not want the led to use their brains. Don't let them stop you: If you have a brain—use it.

18.1 External Success and Inner Fulfillment

The right mix between "vita activa" and "vita contemplativa" is ultimately the individual way of being in the world. Everyone has their subjective interpretation of the world and their more or less conscious sense that they give themselves: having hope without deluding oneself could be a goal. Love can also be described as life's longing for itself. It is the connection of selflessness and self-interest, as it is about the continuation of life. On an individual level, it is good to distinguish the following areas: A good life is a sensual and meaningful life. Because meaning makes resilient, resistant. And it consists in the respective life phase of the appropriate personal mix of **external success** and **inner fulfillment**. For this, it is useful to link the three levels of life with each other:

- Interiority and reconnection (questions of meaning, philosophy, religion)
- Exteriority and factual level ("world exploration and improvement")
- Humanity ("The I becomes an I through the You") and ecology

Is religion for me—as an external system of meaning off the shelf—a solution? Only if it can be integrated in a self-syntonic way, not festering like a stake in the flesh. But—always consider that you could be wrong: "Insanity is the inability to doubt," once said Peter Ustinov.

"Trust those,
who seek the truth.
Not those,
who claim to have found it."

18.2 Interchangeability of Religions

Undoubtedly, religions are transient, but the spiritual primal ground, the infinite source, the flow of energy (or whatever you want to call it) is eternally constant.

"The world would probably
be in a better state,
if stupidity hurt."

The religious contents and images of God are interchangeable between all religions. One could say: The true faith is in the hearts and minds of the believers. And if it is not there, then it is nowhere. External rituals, prayers etc. can be helpful for this, as long as they have an inner meaning for the believer—but without guarantee that they really work. The certainties of today are (perhaps) already the delusions of tomorrow. A consolation is: The truth sometimes goes under—but it does not die. Learning to live with this uncertainty is a piece of art of living: "Thinking instead of praying" could be a good motto.

18.3 Transnihilism

"Believe nothing because a wise man said it.
Believe nothing because everyone believes it.
Believe nothing because it is written.
Believe nothing because it is considered holy.
Believe nothing because another believes it.
Only believe what you yourself have recognized as true."
(Buddha)

More and more people apparently no longer want or need the traditional and predetermined images and rituals. In modern terms, this attitude could be called "Transnihilism", that is, religion without fixed symbols, without cult, without mystery. Perhaps we are eternal pilgrims, searching for ourselves: You are closer to God when you ask a question than when you give an answer. Because the beneficial thing about religion is not **what** you believe, but **how** you believe. And the path to what I consider my true faith may be full of dead ends, full of errors and confusions. Allow yourself to make mistakes on this path: After all, the world is big enough for everyone to be wrong (in their own way).

Especially in times of current consciousness turbulence, man is in constant change. He probably has no fixed core, no lasting "I", but he is constantly changing. If he is successful today, failure may be very close. Depending on the intensity of the (more or less self-determined) life we lead ("No risk, no fun"), we may be a shining hero today and a tragic figure tomorrow. We are all wanderers between our emotional states—between sorrow and anger, between joy and equanimity. It is helpful to occasionally put oneself in the role of the observer and the uninvolved "witness", who looks at what happens to him every day and what he does with his lifetime with a friendly ironic attitude. Even though this is easier said than done, because it requires a lot of psychological energy, it is worth trying from time to time: Carpe diem—seize the day.

"Tear up your plans.
Be smart and stick to miracles.
They have long been recorded
in the grand plan.
Chase away fear
and the fear of fears."
(Mascha Kaléko)

18.4 Future of Religions: Digital Eternity?

Surely is—the history of religions is far from being fully told. The secrets of God will continue to remain unexplored. The traditional religions are old answers to eternal questions. Don't we need new answers to new questions in the 3rd millennium?

If man is "the eye of evolution," as Aldous Huxley writes—what will happen to religions? Will the religions of the future make humans into **"Homo Deus"**(God-men) as predicted by Yuval Noah Harari, the Israeli historian, where something like immortality arises through artificial intelligence, brain upload, because we all become transhumanist cyborgs, where man and machine merge, who then rule the world as demigods? Will we not only live in a Universe in the future, but in a "Multiverse", i.e. in many worlds at the same time?

Or will the machines originally developed by humans eventually take over all power in the world and dictate to us how we should live and what we should think? Will the algorithms of computer programs dictate a standardized worldview to us from which we can no longer escape? Will everything that happens then be recorded and stored into digital eternity?

A similarly structured world was described by Aldous Huxley a hundred years ago in his science fiction novel "Brave New World": a clearly planned and structured life in which individuality is only possible within the given biological and psychological grids and the entire life—from the cradle to the grave—is predetermined and runs like a computerized washing program, where questions of meaning no longer play a role and even individual death is factored in?

Probably (and hopefully) it is still a long way off until the world and the cosmos end in the "Big freeze" (the big freeze), the "Big rip" (the big bang) or the "Big crunch" (the big collapse). Even though we are fortunately not yet that far, a few basic philosophical and religious questions arise for us today:

What remains of us? Is there life after death? The more important question is probably: Is there life before death? Whether after death as a personal identity after the Last Judgment, transformed in another form in the process of reincarnation, whether in the hereafter as a soul being or simply in the material transformation of energy—one thing can be said with certainty: It continues.

"Things are not as they are.
They are always what
one makes of them."
(Ludwig Mies van der Rohe)

References

Korp, Harald-Alexander: Dem ruhigen Geist ist alles möglich, Gütersloh 2019 (Gütersloher Verlagshaus)

Kröger, Fritz: Intelligenz jenseits der Logik, Berlin 2021 (Edition Estrany)

Schweid, Richard: Sehnsucht nach Unsterblichkeit, Gütersloh 2008 (Gütersloher Verlagshaus)

Schmidt-Leukel: Wahrheit in Vielfalt, Gütersloh 2019 (Gütersloher Verlagshaus)

Volf, Miroslav: Zusammen wachsen – Globalisierung braucht Religion, Gütersloh 2017 (Gütersloher Verlagshaus)

Zohar, D. Marshall, I.: SQ – Spirituelle Intelligenz, Bern/München/Wien 1999 (Scherz)

19

Small Lexicon of Esoteric, Religious-spiritual and Philosophical Basic Terms

Summary
This chapter explains and defines the most important terms in the field of religion, religiosity, spirituality, and metaphysics: Since the afterlife is quite confusing, there are a multitude of terms such as spirituality, esotericism, transcendence, metaphysics, atheism, agnosticism, pantheism, polytheism, scientism etc., which are described and explained here.

Definitions

Agnosticism = Philosophical view that nothing can be said about God because he cannot be recognized. Neither the existence nor the non-existence of a higher being is provable according to the agnostic viewpoint.

Animism means that both living beings and inanimate objects have a soul. It is also referred to as "universal animation".

"Antinomy": Two equally well-founded statements are in logical contradiction to each other.

Asceticism: Strictly abstinent lifestyle, with which the individuals try to intensify their spiritual consciousness.

Atheism = Atheists deny that there is a (personal) God or a higher being.

Bible: Holy book of Christians (Old and New Testament).

God's ground staff: Priest, pastor, guru, Brahmin, medium, shaman (see each there).

Book religions = Judaism, Christianity, Islam, as their faith is laid down in the Holy Scriptures (Torah, Bible, Quran).

Chassidism: Spiritual branch of Judaism, which emphasizes the strict interpretation of Jewish laws.

Deism = The view that God created the world but has no further influence on it. (Was particularly represented in the 17th and 18th centuries.).

Dogmatism describes a rigid and unyielding adherence to certain dogmas and beliefs. New perspectives and other perspectives are not allowed. In religion and philosophy, dogmatism is used to describe a narrow-minded attitude that resists any kind of questioning or critical examination of one's own beliefs. Dogmatism is often a negative trait that can lead to intellectual stagnation and prevent people from learning new things and developing.

Jihad: Holy war by Muslims with a religious goal. On the external level, it is a fight against the unbelievers and their conversion. On the internal level, it is a struggle for spiritual development, intellectual progress, and the cultivation of one's own instinctiveness.

Eschatology: Doctrine of the end of times or the totality of religious ideas about the Last Things, i.e., the final fate of the individual and the world.

Esotericism: Originally, esotericism was understood as a kind of spiritual-philosophical secret doctrine. By its word meaning, esotericism means "belonging to the inner area", "understandable from within". Esoteric knowledge was supposed to be accessible only to a limited group of people ("initiates"). (Contrast: Exoteric = generally accessible knowledge). Today, the secret teachings are open to anyone who is willing and able to pay for them. Today, esotericism encompasses all kinds of views and methods that practice and spread their truths outside of traditional religions (spirit healers, fortune tellers, secret masters, etc.). Because today, esotericism draws from a pool of various worldviews and human images -whatever can be sold as new and revolutionary as a "crash course to enlightenment". Esotericism has become a huge business field, in which all sorts of things are offered and sold as miraculous healing practices—from astrology, reincarnation and channeling to gemstone therapy, Native American ear candles, sound bowl massage to levitation and light nutrition. The term esoteric is now used rather pejoratively and is synonymous with many for incomprehensible, spun and charlatanism.

Eucharist: Christian ceremony intended to commemorate the Last Supper of Christ with his disciples. Bread and wine are the central sacred elements. While Catholics believe that the bread and wine are the true body and blood of Christ (transubstantiation), Protestants understand the Eucharist as merely a remembrance of the Last Supper (consubstantiation).

Gospel (= good news): The books of the New Testament (Matthew, Mark, Luke, John)

Evolution is a process by which (biological) species change over generations through natural selection, mutations, and genetic drift. This process is initially undirected and leads to organisms that are better adapted to their environment, thereby improving the survival chances of species. The theory of evolution is widely scientifically proven and is considered a theory that has greatly shaped our view and understanding of the world.

Spirit/Soul: Metaphysical part of a person, which, according to many religions, brings the body to life, supplies it with life force, and continues to live after the death of the body.

Belief: Being convinced of a belief system or dogma that is ultimately not (or only very difficult) to prove.

Gnosis (knowledge): 1st/2nd century AD—ancient movement that draws from Greek philosophy and oriental religions. Strictly dualistic worldview. The otherworldly light world created by God, this worldly, bad world created by "Demiurge". Christ is not a "savior", but only the announcer of the path to salvation. He was not a true human. Self-salvation is possible through "spark of spirit".

God: According to religious philosophers, God is undefinable ("The God that exists does not exist"), but descriptions of him can be found everywhere: the highest, almighty, omniscient, eternal, uncreated, and supernatural being that is not really comprehensible (nameless and indescribable). He is the ruler of the universe, creator of worlds, and director of worlds. In monotheism (see there), God is the personalized embodiment of good, natural force, and moral-spiritual power. For many philosophers, God is rather a principle and thus the basis on which reason ultimately stumbles (for more on this, see: systems of meaning).

Deity: In polytheistic religions, **a** god or a sacred being that embodies certain spiritual qualities or life forces (in Hinduism: e.g., Ganesha = success, Krishna = joy of life, Saraswati = wisdom).

Idol: Derogatory term for a pagan deity of the false or unbelievers.

Guru (word meaning: enlightened, wise, master): Religious teacher who (especially in Hinduism) is regarded by his students as the embodiment of a divine being.

Hadith: Collection of deeds and sayings of the Prophet Mohammed, compiled through oral reports, which (alongside the Quran) forms the basis of the Islamic way of life (see also: Sharia).

Sacred/Sacred: The term sacred (or sacral) refers to something that has high significance, is inviolable or very important, and is respected. If it is linked to religion, it may even be considered significant and revered for moral or ethical reasons. Most religions have sacred texts and books (Bible, Quran, Vedas, Torah…), symbols and places (churches, mosques, synagogues, temples…), rituals and practices (prayers, meditations, mantras, chants). Throughout human development, almost all cultures have had some things or objects that were particularly valuable, meaningful, or "sacred" to the respective people. In some form, a distinction was always made between the *sacred* (or sacral) area and the *profane* (or worldly) area. The sacred often belonged to another world (the hereafter).

Homo religiosus: (Latin for religious man). This term describes people who are deeply devoted to religious belief systems, convictions, and rituals. Religion is an indispensable part of their identity.

Humanism: Attitude that emphasizes the value and dignity of humans

Iconoclasm: Abolition and destruction of holy images, iconoclasm

Imam: Islamic prayer leader in the mosque

Intelligent Design (ID): This is the view of conservative Christian "creationists" (especially in the USA) that certain circumstances in the universe and on Earth can only be explained by an "intelligent originator" (namely God) and not by evolutionary concepts such as natural selection or mutation. Most scientists consider ID to be pseudoscience.

Consubstantiation: The Protestant doctrine of the Eucharist. It emphasizes (in contrast to Catholic transubstantiation) that believers take the body and blood of Christ "in, with, and under" the bread and wine.

Quran: Holy book of Islam

Kosher: Following the rules of Jewish dietary laws

Creationism: According to this concept of conservative Christians in the USA, the origin of the universe, life on earth, and humans occurred exactly as described in the Bible. Strict creationists even claim that the world is only a few thousand years old and that humans and dinosaurs lived on the earth at the same time. In science, creationism is considered pseudoscience (see also: Intelligent Design).

Mahdi: Expected savior in (Shiite) Islam (see also Messiah)

Medium: Person who establishes a connection to spirits, deities, and paranormal forces—or at least claims to do so. Many mediums consider themselves a link or channel ("Channel") between living people and supernatural beings.

Messiah ("Anointed One"): Expected savior (of the Jews). Redeemer, who came into the world for Christians through Jesus.

Metaphysics: Metaphysics (word meaning = beyond physical nature) deals with the fundamental (scientific) truths and their spiritual dimension, the nature of being. Main areas: Universal science (essential scientific principles), ontology (nature of being), and theology (existence of God).

Monotheism: Belief that there is only one (personal) God. Judaism, Christianity, and Islam are the main monotheistic religions. Contrast: Polytheism (polytheism) and Pantheism (God is in everything, the entire nature, the cosmos).

Myth: This is a philosophical-religious narrative about the origin of the world, the cosmos, humans, God, and gods. The term is derived from the ancient Greek word for narrative, legend. Originally, myths were passed on orally until the development of written language. The oldest written myth is the Epic of Gilgamesh. When several myths belong together, we speak of a mythology. Some people therefore refer to religions as mythologies and/or narratives.

Different types of myths can be distinguished:

- Cosmological myths deal with the origin of the world
- Theological M. describe the world of gods
- Anthropological M. explain the origin of humans
- Eschatological M. deal with the end of the world
- Etc.

People interpret the world and their own lives through myths in symbolic stories. Myths are explanatory patterns and often relate to fundamental and existential questions (meaning of life, life after death, good and evil …) and are therefore strongly emotionally charged. Because myths have the psychological and social sense of making inexplicable processes explainable, they are considered to be meaningful

Mysticism: The word "mystical" is often understood in everyday language as "mysterious", "incomprehensible" or "enigmatic". However, there is a mystical dimension in all religions. The goal of mysticism is unification with a higher power (or instance) or immersion in God. In this context, religious externals (rituals, prayers, services, dogmas, etc.) are secondary, as they are used at best as tools to achieve the mystical state. Often, the mystic experiences dogmas as a constraint from which he seeks to free himself. Some mystics are therefore persecuted as heretics (not only in Christianity), some are declared saints (see below). The mystic is concerned with his very subjective-personal relationship with his God ("Unio Mystica"). The mystical path is emotional and experience-oriented. Sometimes ecstatic ("happy") experiences ("expansion of consciousness", 'breakthrough into another reality", "enlightenment") are sought and reported. These experiences are usually very intense, but short-lived. Mystical experiences are usually all-encompassing and paradoxical. They are intuitive and often associated with an "oceanic feeling". The tenor is: "All is one" (Unio Mystica). It is difficult to put mystical experiences into words. Lao-Tse says: "Those who say it do not know. Those who know do not say it." In the Christian context, it would be called "silentium mysticum". It is also not easy to develop a mystical lifestyle from this intense faith experience. In Christianity, Meister Eckhart, Johannes Tauler, Teresa of Avila, Hildegard of Bingen, Ignatius of Loyola, Francis of Assisi, etc. are known as mystics.

Nepotism: Procurement of advantages (e.g., transfer of church offices) to family members or friends

Nihilism: Literally: "Belief in nothing". Questioning of all previous belief, value and meaning systems. Nihilism is a philosophical direction that holds the belief that life has no objective meaning and purpose. All moral and ethical beliefs are, according to the nihilistic view, man-made and changeable. It is a denial or relativization of all beliefs and ideologies. In this thought system, there is neither a God nor any other higher instance. Nihilism is a central motif of existentialism. Moral and ethical beliefs therefore have no fundamental justification. Nihilism is a philosophical direction that questions the existence of God, but also of truths and values.

Numinous: Incomprehensible, trust and fear arousing power of the divine

Pandeism: God created the entire universe and is one with it. He is not a separate being, but has become nature and therefore does not need to be worshipped. (Pandeism combines pantheism and deism.)

Pantheism: Everything is divine and God is in everything.

Pantheon: Temple dedicated to the Roman gods

Pastor: In the Catholic Church, a pastor is a priest who does not lead a parish, but is commissioned by the bishop with other tasks (e.g., pastoral care).

In the Protestant Church, the term pastor is used mainly in Northern and Central Germany for priests who lead congregations.

Pfaffe: Derogatory term for priest

Pfarrer: In the Catholic Church, only a priest can accept a parish post ("Pfarrei"), i.e., be a pastor and take over the leadership of a community. Pfarrer is probably derived from Pfarr-Herr, i.e., the lord of the parish.

Polytheism: Belief that there are several gods/deities, which usually represent different aspects of nature. Polytheism is found in many nature religions, Hinduism, Taoism, Confucianism, etc.

Predestination: This is the idea that God has predetermined everything (including the life of each individual). The opposite pole: free will and the responsibility of each individual.

Priest: In many religions, priests are considered intermediaries between God and man. They act as bearers of a religious (church) office, which is endowed with special divine powers. In the Christian context, they have received a ritual (liturgical) consecration, which authorizes them to perform special cultic actions (e.g., services, baptisms, weddings, funerals).

Reformation: Revolutionary movement that founded the Protestant Church as a split from the Catholic Church. It began in 1517 with the 95 theses that Martin Luther nailed to the Wittenberg Church.

Reincarnation: The concept that the human soul is continually reborn and embodies itself in different entities. In the wheel of life "Samsara", the soul is reborn until it has rid itself of all sins, to completely dissolve in "Nirvana". This view is mainly prevalent in Eastern religions (Hinduism, Buddhism, Jainism).

Religiosity: There is no universally valid definition of religiosity. Religiosity often stems from the desire for meaning, explanation of the world, the attempt to trace unexplainable phenomena back to an understandable cause.

Religiosity belongs to the complex neurobiological phenomena. It is probably not genetically anchored, but most people probably have the ability to develop a "transcendent sense". Religious people believe in a transcendent power, greater than themselves, which—because it stands above them in their belief—provides security and guides their thinking, feeling, and actions. However, this power is not (completely) understandable, explainable, and provable. It can be the belief in a personal God or a force that gives structure, order, and meaning to life (e.g., Tao, Brahman, Evolution, Chi). This is often associated with reverence for the diversity and order of the world and the cosmos, in which believers feel trustingly embedded. Also, belief in this universal power is often associated with religiosity. Highly religious people align their experiences, thinking, feeling, and actions with their faith and try to implement this faith in everyday life. Some have an intrinsic desire for "enlightenment", "transcendence" or "expansion of consciousness".

Religiosity is usually about individual faith experience and faith practice, which focuses on the intrapsychic processing of the external belief system *("on the inner stage")*. This form of R. is called *intrinsic religiosity*.

In contrast, it is called *extrinsic religiosity* when people become religious to gain personal advantages (membership in a religious community, status). Some also call this hypocrisy.

Intrinsic religiosity can be associated with a high emotional charge *(e.g., strong reactions to attacks),* as it is often connected with the core of the personality ("basic trust"). In the various stages of life—from the cradle to the grave—religiosity can have very different meanings (for more on this see Fowler, J. W.: The Stages of Faith. Gütersloh 1991). Religiosity is primarily distinguished from piety (which strongly adheres to external dogmas), hypocrisy (only religious facade), and neurotic religiosity (where religiosity is part of a mental illness).

Sacrament: Ritual action through which God is supposed to act in a special way ("holy mystery"). In the Catholic Church, there are seven sacraments (Baptism, Eucharist/Communion, Confirmation, Penance, Marriage, (Priest-)Ordination, Anointing of the Sick/Last Rites). Among Protestants, there are only two sacraments (Baptism and Communion).

Shaman: Holy persons, who exist mainly in tribal cultures. Although the term originates from Siberia, it is now mainly associated with the Indians. A shaman (man or woman) was/is a spiritual leader in many indigenous peoples. He/she sees himself/herself as a mediator ("medium") between the physical and the supernatural/spiritual world or wants to be their mouthpiece. Many shamans claim to possess and/or channel ("channel") supernatural powers and to be able to heal diseases. In the modern esoteric scene, many consider themselves shamans.

Sharia: Rules and customs by which Islamic life is regulated (see also: Quran and Hadith)

Scholasticism: In the Middle Ages, the Christian Church largely determined the worldview not only of ordinary people but also of the science and philosophy of the time. Influenced mainly by the Dominicans Albertus Magnus and Thomas Aquinas, scholasticism was one of the most important schools of thought in the Middle Ages. It was about the subordination of science and philosophy to the authority of Christian theology: it was only supposed to be scientifically provable what fit into the framework of Christian faith, as it was represented at the time. Anselm of Canterbury coined the phrase "Credo ut intelligam" (I believe in order to know).

The "auctoritates" were the basis of the scholastics' research—i.e., texts from inviolable religious authorities who had contributed to the self-understanding of the Christian faith, such as Church Fathers (Augustine), natural philosophical works of ancient authors (Aristotle), etc. Thomas Aquinas, one of the most important theological authorities in the late Middle Ages, created the working method of dialectics for this purpose. In the "resolutio" of the cognition process, the "true standpoint"—the only valid and binding truth—was then proclaimed, which had to be reconciled with the Christian tenets of faith. However, the scholastics also dealt with more or less absurd questions of faith—e.g., how many angels can fit on the head of a pin?

As the world became increasingly complex, many were no longer satisfied with the reference to divine creation, they wanted to know more about the laws of nature and "what holds the world together". And this brought the sciences to flourish. Many scientists no longer wanted to submit to the church's faith guidelines and questioned them (Copernicus, Galileo). Thus, the sciences became a competitor to the Christian faith.

Schism: Separation of different religious factions in Christianity.

Eastern Schism: Separation of the Roman Catholic from the Orthodox Church (1054). **Western Schism** (1378–1417): During this time, there were several antipopes who resided simultaneously in Rome and Avignon.

Meaning: Man is a being in need of meaning. He wants to know where he comes from, where he is going, what he is supposed to do here. Most want to understand who they are, how the world, the cosmos works, and whether they have a choice ("free will"). What they can know and what they must believe.

Systems of Meaning: This refers to a complex network of values, inner convictions, norms, and goals. With this, man can understand and structure his world and put his experiences into a meaningful context, thus finding meaning, gaining orientation and support. Religion, philosophy, science, art, social, politics, etc. can be sources of these systems of meaning. The individual assembles his individual system of meaning from various areas (more or less consciously), which harmonize with each other or may also conflict with each other. Systems of meaning are not immutable, but they change over the course of a lifetime with the experiences that the person makes throughout his life.

Spirituality: There is no universally valid definition of spirituality. The term is derived from Spiritus (breath, spirit) or Spiro ("I breathe"). Spirituality is a complex construct, but it always assumes that there is more than what we can perceive with our senses (transcendence). In the present, the term is equated with postmodern religiosity (see there). In the Christian area, S. is often equated with piety. However, spirituality can also be lived completely independently of traditional religions. Some also define it as the "search for the sacred".

Fall of Man: Since God had forbidden Adam and Eve to eat a fruit from the tree of knowledge, but they succumbed to the temptation to do so, they were driven out of paradise.

Synchronicity (by C. G. Jung): An inner and an outer event occur simultaneously. However, there is no direct connection. In subjective experience, however, there is a connection, for example, the external event is experienced as a reflection of the inner state.

Syncretism: Merging and fusion of different (aspects of) religions.

Scientism = Belief in science

Talisman: A small object that one carries with oneself and believes to have magical properties, protecting the wearer from injuries, diseases or the "evil eye" and perhaps granting special powers. Often these are pieces of jewelry that are magically-emotionally charged by the person concerned.

Taoism: "Teaching of the way", Chinese philosophy and worldview. The way is the goal: desirelessness, "Wu wei" (letting happen).

Teleology is a philosophical concept that assumes that natural processes, phenomena, and objects were created and oriented for a specific purpose and towards a goal. In dogmatic-Christian theology, there is the view that God created the world and the universe exactly as he wanted ("Intelligent Design", see there). God also created humans in this world exactly as he wanted and—according to this view—has a special focus on them. Teleological views were accepted by Christian science for many centuries. Today, teleology is mostly replaced at the scientific level by evolutionary concepts, according to which the development of species occurs through natural selection and random mutations (without a predetermined purpose) (see also: Evolution).

Theism = God is the creator of the cosmos and the world, who also sustains them and intervenes in them in a guiding manner.

Theodicy: Why does an omniscient and omnipotent God allow so much evil in the world?

Torah: Holy book of the Jews. The first five books of the Old Testament (Genesis, Exodus, Leviticus, Numbers, Deuteronomy) are the basis of the Jewish Bible. They are believed to have been dictated to Moses by God on Mount Sinai and contain instructions for the Jewish faith and all of Jewish life (613 commandments, Mitzvah).

Totemism is the belief in the supernatural power of a totem. A totem is an animal, plant, or inanimate being that is used (partly still today among indigenous peoples) as a tribal sign and is revered. It is often magically and emotionally charged and symbolically represents an (original) ancestor or relative of a people or clan.

Transubstantiation: According to the Catholic Church, doctrine of the Eucharist, the essence of bread and wine transforms into the blood and body of Jesus Christ, but remains in its outward form.

Transcendence: (lat.: going beyond the horizon) Concept according to which it is understood that there are areas of reality that are beyond our everyday experience and can only be grasped to a limited extent with our reason. In religion and philosophy, transcendence is understood as the overcoming of human limitations and access to higher realities. In mystical experiences, an attempt is made to achieve a higher consciousness and/or unity with God or higher powers ("oceanic feeling"). But also in other areas of life (art, music, mathematics, etc.), transcendence describes the exceeding and overcoming of human abilities and extraordinary achievements are sought.

Ubiquity: Doctrine of the Lutherans of the omnipresence of the body of Christ (important for the Protestant doctrine of the Eucharist).

Immaculate Conception: In Christianity, the dogma that Mary, the mother of Jesus, conceived and gave birth to her son "without blemish/sin" ("Immaculata"). In addition, she is also said to have remained a virgin after the birth ("virgin birth"). Thus, she is said to have remained free from original sin.

Vulgate: Latin Bible translation by Church Father Jerome

GPSR Compliance

The European Union's (EU) General Product Safety Regulation (GPSR) is a set of rules that requires consumer products to be safe and our obligations to ensure this.

If you have any concerns about our products, you can contact us on

ProductSafety@springernature.com

In case Publisher is established outside the EU, the EU authorized representative is:

Springer Nature Customer Service Center GmbH
Europaplatz 3
69115 Heidelberg, Germany

www.ingramcontent.com/pod-product-compliance
Lightning Source LLC
LaVergne TN
LVHW010340260326
834688LV00036B/805